WELL-LEADER
MINDSET

OPTIMIZE YOUR HEALTH & WELLNESS ROI

WELL-LEADER MINDSET

Step Into Your Authentic Wellness

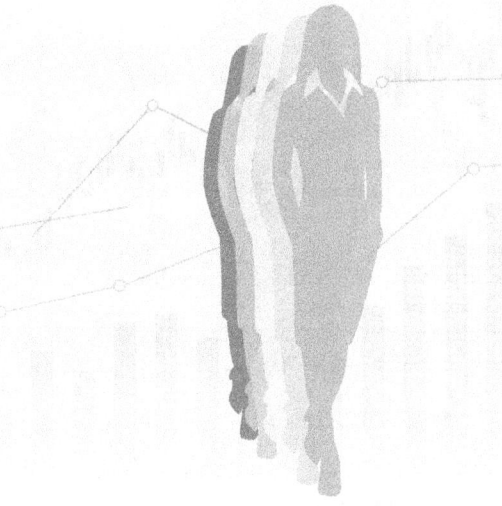

LORI LINDBERGH
PhD, RN, NBC-HWC, DipACLM

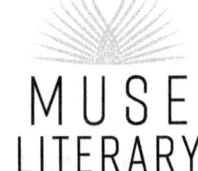

MUSE
LITERARY

Chicago • New York • Rome • Paris

Printed in the United States of America

Hardcover ISBN: 978-1-958714-67-6
Paperback ISBN: 978-1-958714-68-3
Ebook ISBN: 978-1-958714-69-0
Library of Congress Control Number: 2022948339

CHICAGO·NEWYORK·PARIS·ROME

Muse Literary
3319 N. Cicero Avenue
Chicago IL 60641-9998

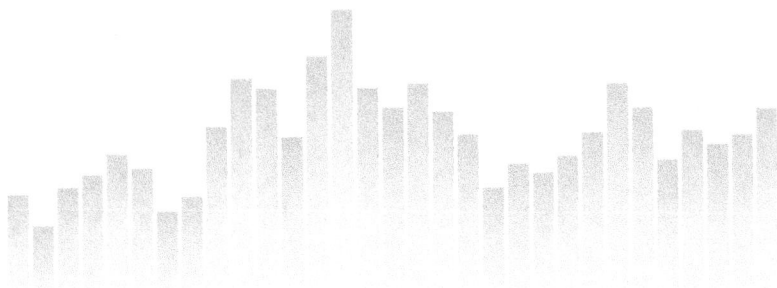

Dedicated in memory of my resilient, WWII Veteran father who inspired my journey; my mother who supported his wellness journey and who still today trusts me with her care and wellness; my husband, David, who is my co-pilot in life and my wellness journey partner and who has always encouraged me to be authentic, extraordinary, and strive for endless possibilities; and my life-changing dog, Luna, for providing her incredible presence and "Lunergy" to keep me going every day, so I get to become the hero of my own journey, share my health and wellness movement with the world, and change countless lives.

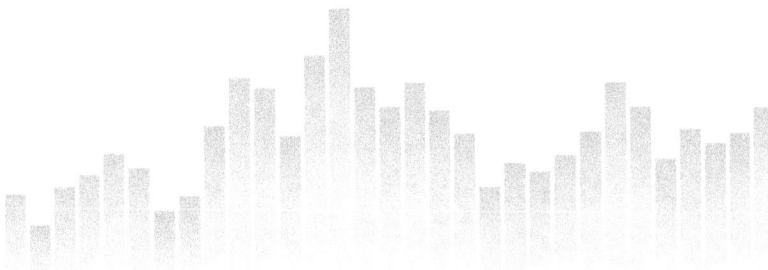

"Wise is wonderful, but probably sets the bar too high. We could be both healthy and wealthy—or at least exercise comparable control over both—if we were just comparably sensible about both health and wealth. Let's give it a try, shall we?"

– Dr. David L. Katz

"No problem can be solved from the same level of consciousness that created it."

– Albert Einstein

"Nothing looks as good as healthy feels."

– Peggy Larson

Disclaimer

The author is providing information to assist you with improving your personal health and wellness. It is up to you to use your own judgment before applying any information and suggestions in your life. The author is not guaranteeing specific results and is not responsible for you misapplying this information in your life. The author is an Industrial-Organizational Psychologist, Registered Nurse, Certified Lifestyle Medicine Professional (DipACLM), Mayo Clinic Certified Wellness Coach, and National Board-Certified Health & Wellness Coach (NBC-HWC), and is not a medical doctor, therapist, or counselor, and is not giving medical or mental health advice or recommendations.

It is your responsibility to always seek medical advice and discuss all health, nutrition, and medical concerns with your physician and/or licensed counselor before you implement any changes. The information presented and evidence-based standards are based on research, books, and publications aligned with the American College of Lifestyle Medicine's (ACLM) evidence-based standards and guidelines, current as of this publication date, and best practices and standards provided by the Mayo Clinic Wellness Coach Training Program and the National Board for Health & Wellness Coaching. The lifestyle wellness strategic planning process and theoretical model of chronic disease progression are proprietary to this author and provide helpful information and guidance to align and support your authentic strategic wellness journey. The model is currently being researched and evaluated by the author.

The lifestyle wellness strategic planning process and theoretical model presented are not in any way a substitute for the advice of your own physician or other licensed medical professionals. Implementing this process worked for this author to optimize her health and wellness return on investment. She is sharing her journey and the experiences of others to illustrate how this process might be helpful for you, too. The author does not guarantee future results or improvement in health status. Your results may vary and are always dependent upon you completing the process fully and implementing the actions and tactics in your life. You should consult your physician and/or medical professionals for further advice on your medical, health, dietary, exercise, or other assistance or advice before implementing actions created as part of this process.

Contents

PART 3
YOUR NEW LIFE TO LIVE

Introduction: It Starts With a Wake-Up Call

You know the feeling: the constant tug of war between knowing you "should" make the healthy choice but choosing the easy, unhealthy default option instead. The feelings you have about your choice and the impact on your current health and wellness may range from frustration, disgust, fear, hopelessness, and helplessness, to even resignation and surrender. As successful leaders and entrepreneurs, we know resignation and surrender are nearly impossible to accept. Those words are not in our vocabulary. We want to be strong, driven, decisive, and supportive for the people in our charge. We put others' needs and our company's needs before our own, we work long hours, we take on way more than we can manage, we bring work home with us, and then rinse and repeat! You see it all happening in real time. You hear the voice in your head saying, "I know I need and *want* to make changes to get healthy, or else." Or else, what? Exactly! You have no idea what to do next. You may have resigned yourself to thinking your current health and wellness is your fate. Maybe this is as good as it gets. You might be right. A statistic cited by the American College of Lifestyle Medicine, reports that only *3% of adults in the US practice healthy levels of four critical health behaviors* (non-smoking, healthy weight management, regular movement, and balanced nutrition).[1]

Where are you now? Are you in the 3% or the 97%? Where do you want to be? If you are with the majority, you may be wondering: How can a successful leader fail so miserably with self-care and self-leadership? You will find out that it's a lot easier than you think and that it's all about how you think and what you believe! My hope is that you are reading this book because you are finally tired of struggling with your health and wellness. You are sick and tired of feeling sick and tired. You want

---

[1] Reeves and Rafferty, "*Healthy Lifestyle Characteristics Among Adults in the US*," 854.

better for yourself. You want to show up fully and become a wellness role model for your people—to pay it forward. Are you in the midst of your own health and wellness wake-up call?

My wake-up call occurred on a cold January morning in 2018. On that day, I finally felt that I had had enough of my persistent "wellness cognitive dissonance" getting the better of me. Cognitive dissonance is the state of having thoughts, beliefs, or attitudes that are inconsistent with your behavioral decisions.[2] In short, your behaviors fail to line up with your desired or ideal thoughts, feelings, and values.

My cognitive dissonance was driven by my never-ending, wellness moving target. I had spent most of my adult life struggling with achieving the health and wellness I desired and envisioned. I set personal goals to achieve "it" when I was 30, 35, then 40, and then 50, maybe 55 or 56 ... I always failed, sometimes miserably. My dissonance manifested as feelings of frustration, discomfort, and guilt from never achieving the health and wellness I so desired and worked so hard to achieve. Typically, cognitive dissonance related to health manifests as negative feelings about failing to do certain behaviors in order to achieve your desire. It could also manifest through continually justifying that it's okay that you know what to do, that you should do it, but that you choose not to do it. In either case, it messes with us, causing psychological stress and even self-sabotage ... as if we leaders need more self-imposed stress and obstacles.

It was different for me. My cognitive dissonance manifested as thinking I was doing everything that was supposed to be correct—what mainstream media and fitness experts promoted at the time—yet I was still failing to achieve my health and wellness goals. I had joined gyms, tried the grapefruit and low-calorie diets, no carb diets, diet pills, shakes, fasting, 21-day and 60-day workout programs, etc. to no avail. At times I came close by using some of the extreme programs; however, I knew what I was doing was not sustainable in the long term. Crash dieting, drinking diet shakes, taking ten grapefruit pills before every meal to feel full, and exercising two to three hours every day wouldn't last. I was right. After a few months, I was back to square one.

As I advanced in my career and embarked on my leadership journey, I experienced another challenge. Increasing work responsibilities, long days, business travel, and long commutes often forced my health and wellness goals to the bottom of my priority list, creating even more dissonance. For the next twenty years, I allowed this to become my rinse-and-repeat pattern further solidifying my wellness cognitive dissonance.

I grew up a skinny, active kid in a small town in western Pennsylvania. I ate what I wanted and was constantly on the move. I was an athlete in high school and college, playing basketball and volleyball. Wellness was the furthest thing from my mind. My active lifestyle and engagement with life kept me fit and lean. After graduating from college and starting my first *real job* as a registered nurse, the

---

[2] Simply Psychology, "*Cognitive Dissonance.*"

yo-yoing began. Shift work, food abundance, and social events took their toll, but I was able to keep my weight in check with extreme dieting and exercising periods when needed. I lived this yo-yo lifestyle until I entered midlife and things changed.

I can't pinpoint exactly when that was. I reached a point when I "yoed" but was unable to "yo" back, no matter what I tried. My body no longer responded to what had typically worked in the past. I found myself stuck on the unhealthy side of the "yo." I had clothes in my closet ranging from size two to size twelve. I had lost the desire and motivation to engage in the extreme diets and intense exercise regimens I had in the past. I needed a new solution to fit my current level of motivation and my busy lifestyle. If my story sounds familiar, I hope it gives you comfort to know you are not alone. I've worked with and have met plenty of leaders who feel the same way. But there is hope—you don't have to live this way any longer!

I had other moments that felt like wake-up calls; however, I will never forget the day that finally jolted me from my life of wellness cognitive dissonance. As a senior leader at a healthcare technology company, I was attending the company's 2018 annual, week-long retreat focused on employee engagement and education, business development, fun, mindfulness, and wellness. The retreat was located at an upscale hotel with impressive accommodations, a full line of spa and wellness amenities, incredible food, and, of course, a well-known coffee bar in the lobby which I visited often. A vendor wellness event was planned, along with mindfulness and relaxation training every day and biometric and fitness testing. In order for employees to receive 100 percent company-paid health insurance, attendance at the vendor health fair, mindfulness and relaxation training, and biometric and fitness testing events was mandatory.

The fateful moment occurred the morning of day three of the event. I felt alone, even though I was sitting in the bustling hotel lobby near the elevators. Voices and sounds were muffled, my mind still reeling from what I had just heard during my biometric screening and fitness testing sessions. The nurse said, "You have stage-one high blood pressure, your cholesterol is almost 300, your LDL and HDL are abnormal, and your body mass index (BMI) indicates you are borderline overweight. Based on this, you have a low to moderate risk for heart disease." My fitness evaluation had produced similar results. The trainer said, "Your fitness level for some areas is low to average, you are in the lower percentile for flexibility, your cardiovascular recovery rate is average, etc. ..."

Sitting in the lobby replaying both conversations in my head, all I could think was, *Seriously, how could this be? I've been exercising, eating less processed food, eating more fruits and vegetables, and I always try to make healthier choices when I travel.* I thought my weight was okay. I still fit into most of my clothes—sort of (at least the ones that contained spandex). After ruminating for about ten minutes, the voice of reality emerged: "Okay, I'll admit I haven't been the best with my nutrition, have not always been consistent with my exercising, I sit all day at work, and, oh yeah, I love cheese ... and wine ... every night. Did I mention I really love cheese?" Until that moment sitting in the lobby,

I was unaware I was on the verge of transitioning into a ticking time bomb! Or maybe I had already crossed over. The days of the skinny, active kid who could eat and drink whatever she wanted without a health and wellness care in the world were over.

Looking for empathy and affirmation that things weren't as bad as I thought, I called David, my husband of over twenty-five years. He was surprised to hear from me that early in the morning, and, after allowing me to vent and express my concerns and disbelief, he stated what we both might have been thinking deep down, "Maybe we've been fooling ourselves." He was great at that—identifying the bottom line and dragging us back to reality. I realize now that we both had been struggling with the same health and wellness concerns, in our own ways. He assured me that, when I got home, we would figure things out together. There had to be something we could do to turn things around. I ended the call feeling better about things. I tried to forget about the morning's events and enjoy the remaining two days at the retreat. That's what leaders must do: move forward and stay in control, or at least fake it. Yeah, right ...

At the awards dinner later that evening, my wellness cognitive dissonance reared its ugly head again. That was it—I solidified in my mind that it was time to end my dissonance, once and for all, with whatever it took. I *would* find the answer. During cocktail hour, my leader colleagues at the table were joking about their own biometric screening and fitness testing results. John said, "The nurse told me I was prediabetic. That can't be right. I'm only 29 years old—diabetes is for old people."

Carole added, "Yeah, I'm old, I'm 57. They tell me that every year, but I don't listen. When you're gonna die, you're gonna die."

To that, Charles replied, "My parents have diabetes and heart disease. That's my future, so I'm going to live and indulge as long as I can."

And finally, Susan offered, "No worries, that's what medications are for. I have plenty of experience with that." Laughter erupted, and Susan raised her wine glass to propose a toast: "To drugs!" Everyone followed suit, including me, reluctantly. I had listened silently, without volunteering to comment—taking it all in, laughing and smiling so I wouldn't look out of place.

I remember thinking, *what's wrong with this picture?* Here I am at a company retreat with a focus on relaxation, mindfulness, and well-being. The company has an incredible employee wellness program with incentives. Everyone wore fitness trackers and seemed to be checking off the boxes to get their fully paid health insurance. But I was sitting with a group of successful, driven leaders who didn't seem to "give a damn" about the future of their health and wellness. They seemed resigned to accept whatever their health and wellness destinies held. How could we be in control and successful in our professional lives while willingly relinquishing control of our health and wellness to destiny—essentially burying our heads in the sand?

That was my wake-up call, my "*not me*" moment. At that table, I made the decision I was not going to accept this as my fate. Poor health and living with chronic diseases were *not* going to be my destiny.

I made the conscious choice to find a way to end my health and wellness cognitive dissonance—no more inconsistency and disharmony, no more self-imposed psychological stress.

As I had learned more about cognitive dissonance, I found that it wasn't necessarily a bad thing, once you recognized *why* it existed. In my case, it prompted me to decide to make positive changes; I realized I was tired of my actions and beliefs being at odds. However, my leadership colleagues seemed to accept their cognitive dissonance, which led them to rationalize and accept their health status. This acceptance would sustain the attitudes and behaviors that, sadly, would continue to impact their health and lifespan. I knew my cognitive dissonance was and would continue to be a source of stress until I acknowledged it and made the decision to permanently eliminate it.

Acknowledgement, check, but now what? I already felt I had tried everything, but now, in my mid-fifties, I was still struggling. What was left to try? Nothing seemed to work or stick in the long term. I had the support of an organization with an incredible wellness program that provided incentives and encouragement for participation, and I still couldn't figure it out. Like other colleagues, I was actively participating and checking off all the boxes, but similar to other leaders and employees, I was as unhealthy as ever.

About two months after the retreat, after some research and soul searching, I figured out what I needed to do. With my husband's support, I mustered the courage to leave my leadership career behind to pursue my renewed passion for psychology, health and wellness coaching, and lifestyle medicine. Lifestyle medicine is the use of evidence-based approaches to address chronic diseases by replacing unhealthy behaviors with positive behaviors in six areas: healthful eating, increased movement, improved sleep, managing stress, avoiding risky substances, and developing and maintaining positivity and connections.[3] I have combined all these disciplines with my entrepreneurial focus to help busy, successful leaders eliminate their cognitive dissonance by changing their thinking and adopting a more strategic, lifelong investment approach to their health and wellness—one in which they no longer have to accept their destiny of developing chronic diseases and they truly believe they are no longer at the mercy of their genetics. A life in which they feel healthier, younger, and more vibrant using evidence-based, lifestyle medicine practices.

My mission is helping leaders change their thinking and beliefs so they can be well and can "live well and lead well" and empower those in their charge (at home and work) to seek a lifestyle of wellness. That's the essence of my Well-Leader Mindset™ (WLM) strategic wellness progression. I believe wellness starts at the top. Leaders must be role models and *walk the wellness talk* to make a difference and create a true culture of wellness, not only in their personal lives but in their organizations by creating a culture where employees can thrive. The current bottom up, grassroots, employee-led wellness approach is not working. I realize this is quite a lofty mission—or should I say a passionate movement!

---

[3] American College of Lifestyle Medicine, *"What is Lifestyle Medicine?"*

How to Use This Book

This book will be your guide to help you use mindset, strategy, and planning tools and best practices to transform your mindset into that of a Well-Leader. You will apply these tools and practices within the context of your health and wellness, however, you can use these to enhance all areas of your life. You will learn how to think more strategically and long term about how to achieve and maintain the lifelong wellness you desire, believe you can and will do it, and end the wellness cognitive dissonance you may be experiencing. You wouldn't run your business or your department without a strategic plan, would you? Your health and wellness should be no different. It is one of your life's biggest projects, why not design it, plan it, and invest in it your way? I will be here every step along the way as your guide, helping you create an authentic lifetime wellness strategy custom-fit for your busy life. This is the only way to *finally* put an end to your wellness cognitive dissonance!

I will share my journey and the journeys of clients who were where you are now. You must be in it for the long haul and be ready for minor setbacks. It takes courage, confidence, commitment, and practice to change your thinking and align your beliefs so you can step out of your default, put yourself first, and *be okay with it*. It takes time and patience to step back and do the groundwork to create an authentic "Lifestyle Wellness Strategic Plan" that realistically works for your life. This is not a 30, 60, or 90-day thing—this is for life. Your life. I've been transforming my mindset and implementing my own *Lifestyle Wellness Strategic Plan* for over four years. I revisit my plan often to update it and adapt to what life throws my way. "Living Well and Leading Well" is simply what I do. It feels comfortable and effortless. It is within your grasp, too!

This book is *not* a quick weekend read—it takes time to shift your mindset and create a custom wellness plan that works for your life. The planning process you will experience is *intense* and flows more like a college course spread out over a series of weeks, giving you time to read, apply, reflect on your progress, and course-correct as desired. The process aligns with my 12-week Well-Leader Mindset™-Activate program. I've found that it takes practice, coaching support, and time to begin experiencing the mindset shift to change your wellness trajectory. You could complete this planning process sooner; however, fully completing and reflecting on all strategic wellness activities is incredibly important. Your goal should be to complete your plan over twelve weeks, which seems to be the sweet spot for most leaders. I've had clients attempt to shorten or extend the planning period, only to find that work and life as usual get in the way. Unfortunately, they typically end up back where they started. As with any project, spending focused time upfront leads to longer-term success. Quoting my husband's T-7 aphorism, you must, "Take The Time To Take The Time!" As with any important project, failing to plan is planning to fail.

This book is divided into three parts. The chapters in each part build upon the previous chapters' strategic wellness activities. To experience the most value and compile your comprehensive, authentic

Lifestyle Wellness Strategic Plan, work through the chapters sequentially, completing all activities, evaluations, and reflections fully. I've added checkpoints throughout the process for you to reflect on your progress and weigh in on how courageous and confident you are feeling about moving forward. Part 1 helps you build a strong foundation upon which to begin your strategic wellness journey. The chapters in Part 1 build awareness of your current mindset and transform the way you think about change and transformation; they help you truly understand where you are now, uncover the strengths you can leverage to support your journey, and encourage you to dig deep to identify the true, intrinsic reasons why you want to embark on your lifetime journey toward health and wellness. You will develop a vision for the health and wellness you desire and define where you want to go and where you see yourself in the future.

The chapters in Part 2 help you evaluate your *Current Baseline* and determine how far you are willing to go to achieve the health and wellness future you desire and believe is possible for you. Is your goal to implement evidence-based actions that may reverse the chronic diseases of lifestyle you already have, slow their progression, or prevent them from occurring in the first place? You decide. You are always in control. Applying the proprietary process, theoretical model, and evaluation methods included will help you end your wellness cognitive dissonance. This happens by level-setting your expectations about where you desire to go and aligning what it will take to start and maintain your journey toward wellness and beyond—whichever goal you choose.

The chapters in Part 3 dive into the tactical planning process—the nuts and bolts of what will truly work in your life to get you where you want to go. You will learn about evidence-based tactics that have been shown to improve critical components of your health and wellness—actions that have the potential to prevent and reverse chronic diseases of lifestyle. You will set an initial planning horizon of six months—enough time to start at a manageable level and build up to where you see yourself in the future. Overall, I believe the evidence-based, *Lifestyle Wellness Strategic Plan* development process will help you change your thinking to focus on what is possible for you. You will be able to visualize what it will take and how you can easily integrate changes into all areas of your life without feeling as though you are giving up everything and adding more time to your busy schedule. When all is said and done, you will have a personalized *Lifestyle Wellness Strategic Plan* containing all the components that support your successful Well-Leader Mindset™ transformation. Your plan will include a process to evaluate and measure your ongoing success and triggers to ensure you recognize when it's time to adjust. It is all but guaranteed your life will get in the way. You will adjust your initial plan accordingly. This time, however, you will have developed strategies to recognize challenges before they happen and resilience tactics to get you through the bumps in the road.

What You Can Achieve

After years of struggling, I would never have imagined I could achieve the incredible health, wellness, and life clarity that I've achieved now. It seems almost effortless, at least from a psychological perspective—and no more wellness cognitive dissonance. I feel more energetic, engaged, and younger than ever. Sure, I still experience down days. The difference now is that I have the mindset and resilience tactics to fall back on to keep me focused and on track with my wellness journey. I'm sure you want the same. You didn't pick up this book by accident. If you're reading this, it's because you want something better for yourself and you have hope that the health and wellness you desire is possible for you. You don't want to be at the mercy of your genetics any longer.

As a leader, I know you've heard the definition of insanity: doing the same things over and over and expecting different results. It's time to stop the insanity and achieve the health and wellness you desire. I know change is sometimes difficult—especially trying to be healthy in an unhealthy world. I hope that my story will help you see there is a way out and you become inspired to take control of your own health and wellness, not simply hope for the best. You are not alone. I have worked with many leaders who struggle with their health and wellness every day and justify maintaining their poor health by saying, "I will focus on it after this, or that, or when this happens, or when work slows down, or when my kids grow up ..." Now is the time. You don't want to wish next year or after you receive bad news from your doctor that you had started today! This book provides the framework and support for you to embark on your journey toward a better health and wellness future, one in which you may feel younger, more energetic, and live out your life engaged and free from chronic diseases of lifestyle. Think about what may be possible for you!

I'm here and ready to support your strategic health and wellness journey as I have done for many others, so you can truly *live well and lead well*, and inspire others like the leader you were meant to be. Eliminate the health and wellness cognitive dissonance you may be experiencing. No more guilt and negative self-talk or beating yourself up. This time you can be confident you are implementing evidence-based tactics that are truly aligned with the level of health and wellness you envision. There's no need to become an extreme athlete; however, research supports that lifestyle changes may have a dose-response relationship. You must do *enough* to experience the changes you desire. By the end of this wellness strategic planning process, you will know what enough looks like—the level of lifestyle change and associated behaviors that have the potential to support the health and wellness you envision for yourself and believe is possible.

Everything to get unstuck with your wellness and shift your mindset by creating your *Lifestyle Wellness Strategic Plan* is included in this book and the companion *WLM Investment Guide*. Resolving your wellness cognitive dissonance and becoming a savvy wellness investor for life is not a passive experience. The *WLM Investment Guide* is *essential* and *required* to complete the strategic wellness planning process and to "Live and Do" the book. The investment guide contains worksheets, reflections, evaluation tools, planning guides, links, and additional instructions to support you as you work through the strategic wellness activities in each chapter to clarify your next steps toward achieving your authentic health and wellness. I've created a complimentary book resource website at: <u>www.well-leadermindset.com</u> to subscribe to receive weekly strategy emails, download fillable forms, and access videos and helpful resources. Also, join my LinkedIn group: Well-Leader Mindset™—The 3% Club for ongoing support, additional resources, and to collaborate with other Well-Leaders as you embark on your wellness mindset transformation. Do you have the courage and confidence to take control of your thinking and become a Well-Leader? Are you ready to take control of your health and wellness and choose prevention over convention? When you do take control, you can and you will step into your authentic wellness—the wellness that you decide feels right for you. Let's get started!

Strategic Wellness Activities

You've made a critical decision to take the time to *focus on you* for the next twelve weeks as you begin your wellness journey of a lifetime. You get to transform your mindset into one that *believes* and *supports* achieving the health and wellness you desire is possible!

1. **Procure your companion *WLM Investment Guide* and access the book resource website.**
   The essential guide contains detailed instructions and worksheets for the strategic wellness activities, your *Lifestyle Wellness Strategic Plan* template, and space for journaling, reflective writing, and space for responding to checkpoint questions. Access the book resource website at <u>www.well-leadermindset.com</u> or use the QR Code below. Enter your email address to receive weekly email support and access to fillable PDF versions of all forms from the guide, should you prefer to complete your plan development work electronically.

2. **Complete the reflective writing activity.**
   You may have had other experiences that felt like wake-up calls, but these experiences didn't motivate you to change or didn't stick. This is normal. What is different this time?

You can experience cognitive dissonance with your health and wellness and in other areas of your life. By working through this program and stepping into your authentic wellness, you can, and you will end your wellness cognitive dissonance. How do you know when it has ended? It ends when you achieve your *authentic health and wellness*. You no longer hear yourself saying (aloud or in thought), "I should..., I shouldn't..., I know this isn't healthy but..., I'm being bad, I'm lazy, etc." Your *authentic wellness* ends the dissonance by aligning your behaviors with the desired wellness that fits your lifestyle. You genuinely believe in and live your effortless new healthy way of life.

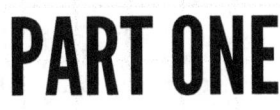

PART ONE

The Beginning of the End of Wellness Cognitive Dissonance

Part 1 begins your journey by guiding you through the process to establish a strong foundation upon which to build your *Lifestyle Wellness Strategic Plan*, focusing on awareness of your thinking and beginning your Well-Leader Mindset™ strategic wellness progression. The first step to any sustained transformation is to develop a baseline, including an understanding of your current self, where you are now, and how your current thinking and behaviors may support or detract from the health and wellness you desire. Completing the readings and strategic wellness activities fully in Part 1 will help you create your lifestyle wellness mission and vision statement based on your "Wellness Why" and "Wellness Vision." This describes your overall, lasting formulation of why you want to embark on your wellness journey and who you hope to be as your best self. Your wellness mission and vision statement paint a picture of where you desire your health and wellness to be in the future. By making your *Wellness Vision* concrete, you will solidify your beliefs and future vision of yourself and use your vision as your beacon, guiding you toward creating a plan that supports your success.

Next, you will identify and engage your core strengths and values, what I call your "Wellness Authenticity," which define the central "musts" and vital principles that will guide you in the day-to-day and long-range decision-making that affects your lifestyle wellness choices. You get to begin leveraging the strengths you already have inside you to change your thinking and enhance your courage and confidence that you can achieve the wellness you desire this time. You will hone your wellness transformation by documenting your strengths to solidify them in your mind and aligning your wellness mission, vision, and aspirations with your strengths. When your *Lifestyle Wellness Strategic Plan* aligns with your strengths, achievement of your best self feels effortless.

Finally, you will focus on building what I call your "Wellness Presence." This includes a current state analysis of your beliefs about your readiness, importance, confidence, and enthusiasm (RICE analysis) about achieving the health and wellness you desire. These four key components can support or derail your strategic wellness journey by affecting your motivation to achieve your best self. Your RICE analysis represents a snapshot of these components and identifies gaps to fill, assets to leverage, and risks you may encounter along the way. Awareness of these components and understanding how they influence your motivation helps you create resilience tactics to keep them at high levels and keep you on track with your wellness when life gets in the way. Combined with your strengths and core values, your RICE analysis highlights the *uniqueness* you get to use to support your belief that you can and you will achieve your best self.

Each chapter in Part 1 builds awareness of your current thinking, helps you truly understand where you are now, uncovers the strengths you can leverage to support your journey, and encourages you to dig deep to identify the true, intrinsic reasons you want to embark on your lifetime journey toward health and wellness. It's time for your mindset to change and for you to gain authority over your own thinking–for you to *believe* that the people who care about you, those you are leading, and those in your personal life, all need you to get your wellness together. Failure is not an option this time. It's never too late to be who you might have been. Start where you are and think about what you can do right now that would feel meaningful and inspire you to embark on your wellness journey. You've taken a great first step, so let's keep the momentum going!

CHAPTER ONE

Give Yourself the Gift of Wellness

You've read how I experienced my wake-up call. You may be at a similar point or feel as if you are getting close. So now what? That's the million-dollar question many people face after experiencing rock bottom. After returning home from the company event, my husband and I spent time brainstorming the answer to that question. What did we come up with? We decided to try a new fitness program and adjust our diet—the same tactical approach we had tried in the past. Remember the definition of insanity: doing the same things over and over but expecting different results. With that in mind, we made sure the new fitness program we implemented was different than before. It was a foundational program focusing on strengthening, relaxation, yoga, and healing from the inside out. Our nutritional program was more aligned with a whole-food, plant-based diet, and I eliminated my nemesis, cheese. We were satisfied that both programs were different enough from what we had tried in the past. However, they were still tactical, not the strategic perspective I now know is required to achieve lifelong health and wellness. I was okay with what we decided to do in conjunction with my search for more answers.

Then one day, it happened: my "aha" moment. I remember that moment like it was yesterday. It happened during one of my marathon Google searches ... the pivotal moment I found my life's passion—always better late than never! I decided then to pursue a career in health and wellness coaching and lifestyle medicine. It wouldn't be a quick path, however. All in, it would take at least two to three years for me to gain the knowledge and experience required to achieve certifications in both disciplines. I made the commitment two weeks later by resigning from my leadership role, enrolling in the Mayo Clinic Wellness Coach Training Program, and never looking back.

It wasn't a difficult decision for me. Thinking about my last leadership role, I knew I had someone's dream job—yet I was usually miserable, tired, and lifeless. I was running on caffeine in the morning, eating what I thought I was supposed to eat to be healthy, and downing a few glasses of wine *every* night to relax. Sound familiar? Through my research, I realized things didn't have to be that way, and that was all I needed. I was ready to embrace new possibilities. Think about how you would feel to know that you may *not* be at the mercy of your genetics when it comes to your health and wellness. That you may *not* be destined to become overweight, develop diabetes, high blood pressure, heart disease, or cancer because it runs in your family. Would you be willing to do what it takes for the rest of your life?

I truly believe that lifestyle medicine practices can prevent and reverse many chronic diseases of lifestyle, even if the diseases run in your family. The evidence supporting this is growing every day. My wish for you—and the reason I wrote this book—is that you decide to take back control of your own life. Improved health and wellness can be your destiny. Since that fateful day sitting around that table listening and watching my leadership colleagues take their health and wellness for granted, I have achieved certification as a Mayo Clinic Wellness Coach, national board-certification as a health and wellness coach (NBC-HWC), and certification by the American College of Lifestyle Medicine as Diplomate for Proficiency and Specialization as a Certified Lifestyle Medicine Professional (DipACLM). I've been able to shrink my growing waistline, I'm feeling stronger, more fit, vibrant, pain-free, and younger than ever, and I've been able to fend off the chronic diseases of middle age (in my genetics) that were beginning to set in. It is as though I've found the fountain of youth. And I've done it all using lifestyle changes. *No* pills or procedures here. I've coached entrepreneurs and leaders in organizations to do the same. It's your turn now!

Throughout this process, I've realized my greatest source of stress was the leadership position I held with a company whose culture was no longer a good fit for me. After I resigned to take care of myself and pursue my health and wellness passion, I experienced a profound sense of relief and optimism. I was ready. It was finally time for me to "give myself the gift of wellness," which was something I valued highly and had never been able to achieve. The amazing thing I found along my journey was that, through my role modeling and excitement, I was able to give the gift of wellness to others directly and indirectly. Those close to me experienced a change in their own wellness and were able to reverse and stop chronic diseases from progressing: my husband, my parents, and two of my sisters.

It's time for me to pass on the gift of wellness to you. Are you open to accepting this mission? You don't have to quit your job to achieve the health and wellness you desire. It's about changing your thinking and finding out what works for you within the context of your own life; your journey is specific to you. Discovery is all part of the journey. Lifelong wellness must fit into your desired lifestyle, not feel like extra time and effort, and not seem as though you are giving up everything you've enjoyed in the past. Once you change your thinking, you can manage your wellness cognitive dissonance by level-setting your expectations about the health and wellness you desire and matching your expectations with your actions to achieve what you envision. You will then be able to make informed decisions and understand the impacts of your decisions on your *Wellness Vision*. You choose your desired health and wellness and create your lifestyle wellness strategy accordingly. Are you ready to feel healthier, more vibrant, and inspire others along the way? Continue reading if your answer is *yes*, *maybe*, or if you are still unsure.

You have the ability to be healthy, feel younger, and experience a renewed sense of well-being in your life, but only *you* can give yourself this gift! It doesn't come in a pill, package, diet bar, fad diet, or a 30-, 60-, or 90-day get-fit-quick program. It comes from within, from what you already have inside yourself! However, living disease-free takes strategic planning. You wouldn't run your business or your department without a strategic plan, would you? Your health and wellness destiny *is* your business. No one else can run it but you. You are the CEO of your own wellness! Creating and implementing a *Lifestyle Wellness Strategic Plan* puts you back in control. Your health and wellness are more important than ever. Your custom plan will help you begin your journey of a lifetime and travel the road to true wellness—one that will help you achieve your best self. You will live a life in which you feel healthier, energetic, and more vibrant, while leading and inspiring others along the way. Become part of the *Well-Leader Mindset™ 3% Club*.

Throughout my leadership wellness coaching, I've met successful leaders who felt stuck in a rut— old, tired, unhealthy, and lifeless ... similar to what I had been feeling. They were essentially living the same year over and over, passively hoping chronic diseases of lifestyle wouldn't set in. I know now that it doesn't have to be this way; however, you need more than hope to fend off lifestyle-related chronic diseases. Like me, many thought they were doing the right things to achieve health and wellness, but nothing seemed to work. You may be having the same thoughts—that you've tried everything to help you feel healthier and more energetic. You may even have accepted that you are destined to feel old, gain weight, or develop diabetes or heart disease, and you have resigned yourself to that, simply letting your genetics run their course. I know I'm beginning to sound like a broken record, but it's time to *think again*! It's time to become a lifelong, strategic health-seeker and choose strategic wellness. If you are reading this book, you know it's *time* to make a choice: Grow old with *health* or grow old with *disease*. Are you ready to make that choice? Regardless of your answer, I encourage you to continue reading with an open, curious mind.

You might be wondering why I keep asking if you are ready. Truly giving yourself the gift of wellness is not for the faint of heart. You may have to blow up some areas of your life to escape and be healthy in an unhealthy world. I've been at it for five years and am still adapting and adjusting to what life throws my way. That's the nature of living a lifestyle of wellness. When you are ready, commit to putting in the effort to change your thinking and discover your desired *future self*, using the evidence-based *Lifestyle Wellness Strategic Plan* development process.

You may still be unsure you have what it takes. I believe you do! This process will help you see that you are truly ready, motivated, and have what it takes to *finally live well and lead well*. As a leader, you are already familiar with the strategic planning process for your organization or department. This book aligns with a strategic planning process for your personal wellness. You will end up with a solid, authentic wellness plan you can easily implement on your own, or you can seek support with implementation and ongoing maintenance and sustainment. The process guides you through the steps to develop the strategic foundation for your successful wellness journey, using a series of strategic wellness activities in each chapter to create the key inputs for your plan. The *WLM Investment Guide* contains easy-to-use worksheets required to complete the planning process, plus additional support on the book resource website at www.well-leadermindset.com.

By the time you reach the end of this book, you will be ready to implement your plan and embark on your lifelong wellness journey. You will have developed your authentic *Lifestyle Wellness Strategic Plan* based on where you are now and how far you are willing to go to believe and achieve your desired health and wellness. Working through the strategic wellness activities will get you started on implementing your plan and experimenting with what works for you to create a life that supports your desired wellness. The focus is on getting your mindset right *first* before reflexively taking action like you (and I) are used to doing. The planning process helps you step back to take a more global, strategic perspective—the perspective I have found leads to lifestyle wellness now and beyond.

Stop putting your self-care on hold. The time is *now*. It's time to change your perspective to one in which you believe your self-care is mandatory, not an indulgence. In today's environment, self-care is not simply a nice thing to have anymore. Staying healthy is a *requirement*, and it *must* become your new way of life. Now that you've made the critical decision to *focus on you* as you begin your wellness journey of a lifetime to transition toward achieving the health and wellness you desire, how does that make you feel? Excited, unsure, resistant, reluctant, nervous, or even just plain scared? You may experience all these feelings throughout your journey, and that is *normal*! Before you dive in full speed like I know you are ready to do, I would like to provide a few tips for success.

1. Any time you start a strategic journey—especially your wellness strategic journey—it is important to plan and prepare to achieve success. *I recommend completing the process presented in this book across twelve weeks.* That's reading one to three chapters per week and completing the strategic wellness activities in each chapter. The *WLM Investment Guide* contains a suggested weekly completion outline. Also, the book resource website is organized by weeks to

keep you on track with your planning activities. *Failing to Plan = Planning to Fail.* When will you make time for strategic wellness planning in your daily schedule?

2. You must *show up* fully to reap the benefits of your *Lifestyle Wellness Strategic Plan* development journey. What does it look like to show up? Not only is making time important, but you must also fully engage in the strategic wellness activities in each chapter. I admit the activities may seem a little quirky and repetitive at times; however, they are evidence-based. There is a method to my madness. Complete all the reflective writing/journaling activities and checkpoints to help you continue to progress your Well-Leader Mindset™. There is space for writing in the guide. Journaling and reflective writing are great ways to visualize your thoughts, feelings, and insights throughout your journey. Think of your thoughts as simply sentences in your head. When you see your thoughts in writing, you can organize, understand, and challenge your own thinking and reasoning throughout the planning process, enhance your knowledge and self-understanding, and broaden your perspective about your strategic wellness journey.

3. Collaborate, ask questions, and share your insights about your progress in my LinkedIn group Well-Leader Mindset™—The 3% Club. Interacting in community provides a valuable opportunity to connect and learn from others, support their journeys, and continue to progress your own mindset.

Showing up for yourself takes place in the actions and behaviors you repeat, often without thinking much about them. The time is now for you to start thinking about the things you do—or don't do—to support your wellness every day. The *Lifestyle Wellness Strategic Plan* development process requires you to consistently show up each week to think about and develop the components of a plan that will work for you as you begin and sustain your lifetime wellness journey. Showing up for your wellness when times are good can be hard enough for busy leaders; showing up for your wellness when you're going through a busy time or rough patch may seem downright impossible. But, of course, that is when you benefit from it the most. As you move through the wellness strategic planning process, you will begin to feel your current normal transition to a new normal—one that supports health and wellness. Your *Lifestyle Wellness Strategic Plan* will help you make a big impact on your life and keep you showing up for your own health and wellness. It all begins with scheduling time to show up for yourself *now*. Start small and go from there.

Strategic Wellness Activities

It's time to commit. How and when do you get to show up for yourself? Just as you do in your work, you must commit the time to achieve the wellness you desire. Think about the best time(s) for you to complete your *Lifestyle Wellness Strategic Plan* development activities. Only you can complete the activities—no delegating this time!

1. **Review your primary calendar.**
   Schedule three-to-five hours per week to read, reflect, and complete each chapter's strategic wellness activities. Document the days/times you commit to completing your planning activities. It works best to have standing appointments each week. You can break your time into smaller chunks if that works better with your schedule. Block off the time on your calendar, color code your wellness appointments with yourself using your favorite color (thanks to one of my clients for this tip), and set reminders. Treat your wellness appointments as essential meetings you get to attend, as you would important business meetings. Don't be a no-show or cancel on yourself. You are worth it!

2. **Plan for work and life getting in the way.**
   Identify one to two techniques you will use to help you stay committed to the time you have blocked off in your schedule. If you have an assistant, ask your assistant to schedule your meetings and support your journey.

3. **Complete the Courage & Confidence Check.**
   It takes courage and confidence to achieve the wellness you desire. Rate your courage and confidence levels with your ability to commit the time and show up for yourself in order to achieve the health and wellness you desire.

4. **Complete the reflective writing activity.**
   Not a fan of journaling or reflective writing? Before you skip this important activity, hear me out. According to critical thinking experts, journaling is an important way to help you visualize and organize your thinking, externalize your thinking, and examine the soundness of your reasoning about a subject or activity.[4] Who would have thought? Many studies show the positive effects of journaling on overall well-being.[5] Journaling offers a safe, confidential, and free way to disclose any thoughts and emotions that may support or may have been getting in the way of your progress toward your best self. Journaling also helps with self-awareness. By turning your attention inward through journaling, you can become more aware of your traits, behaviors, feelings, beliefs, values, and motivations. Becoming more self-aware can increase

---

[4] New York Institute of Technology. "*Developing Critical Thinking With Journal Writing.*"
[5] Ackerman, "*83 Benefits of Journaling.*"

your confidence and can also help you make better decisions aligned with your long-term health and wellness goals. Like any skill, practice leads to improvement. Journaling is no exception. Don't hesitate to add this new, insightful dimension to your self-discovery. One of my clients kept a journal for recording business meeting notes and added a daily wellness entry. Your journal can be a Word document, app on your phone, your guide, or you can go old-school with a notebook. You decide what works for you.

5. **Join my LinkedIn Group Well-Leader Mindset™—The 3% Club.**
   Collaborate with like-minded Well-Leaders. Search for my group or use the link on the book resource website.

   Creating your *Lifestyle Wellness Strategic Plan* will instill in you the courage and confidence to finally believe you can, and you will give yourself the gift of wellness and begin your health journey of a lifetime. I want to warn you, however, that the planning process may feel intense and overwhelming at times. Think about the last offsite strategic planning session or intense project planning session you attended. Strategic planning, regardless of the focus, can feel intense. This is normal even to those who love to plan, like me. You may be tempted to bypass all this planning and just get started *doing*. Resist that temptation! That's the decisive, action-oriented, results-oriented leader in you trying to take control. Taking time to plan your wellness strategy *is* taking action. You must be ready to step back and commit the time to create your *Lifestyle Wellness Strategic Plan*. Anything worth doing that provides lifelong value requires commitment. If not now, when? When you feel you are ready, continue to the next chapter to *seize the movement*!

Dr. Lori's Insights

- New to journaling? Start small and go from there. Start by spending three-to-five minutes writing any thoughts that pop into your head about your wellness journey. There is no right or wrong way to journal; simply do what feels right to you. As with any new skill, it will get easier each time you do it.
- Treat your personal wellness as you would your business. Schedule meetings and appointments to take care of yourself daily, including time to complete the chapter activities throughout the planning process.
- You wouldn't go into a business meeting unprepared, or create an incomplete strategic plan, would you? Prepare to show up for *you* every day!
- To keep wellness in the forefront of your mind (and at the top of your to-do list), review your strategic planning work daily. As you think more about your wellness and move through the

chapters, you will learn new information to help you think differently. This may stimulate new ideas and insights for you to incorporate into your *Lifestyle Wellness Strategic Plan*.

CHAPTER TWO

Seize the Movement!

Committing to an unknown future and stepping out of your comfort zone can be frightening and overwhelming. You experience relief and excitement at first, then feelings of doubt or anxiety may creep in. After my feelings of relief about my own journey subsided, my thoughts about jumping off the career cliff into the deep end turned to anxiety and fear of the uncertain future ahead. I was confident I could do it; however, my self-doubt crept in often, asking, "Do I really have what it will take to pull this off?" Enter my husband, my proverbial cheerleader! Everyone needs a cheerleader. Who is your cheerleader? Every time the doubt crept in, he was there to talk me back down to my reality of possibilities—I *could* do this! I have learned throughout my journey thus far to never underestimate the importance of a supportive spouse, partner, family member, colleague, or friend. Now would be a great time to begin developing your support network—the people who are truly there for you, who will support and encourage you along your health and wellness journey and provide affirmation that you are on the right path. Choose wisely.

You have heard of seizing the moment, but what do I mean by *seizing the movement*? A moment is an exact point in time; a movement is a progressive development over a longer duration and can include a group of people working together to advance a shared campaign. I used *seize the movement* as the title of this chapter to mean: *getting your thinking about your health and wellness unstuck and in your control, so you can move forward collaboratively to achieve your best self.* You do not have to do it alone. You get to have your family, colleagues, support network, and Well-Leader Mindset™ community all working together to advance your own and the collective group thinking about health and wellness. You are becoming a Well-Leader who acts as a role model for wellness, and, in so doing, creates a ripple effect and inspires wellness in others. Definitely a movement, not simply a moment!

I seized my movement by enrolling in the Mayo Clinic Wellness Coach Training Program while concurrently securing a part-time, contractual position as an onsite leadership and employee wellness coach: check and check. After having been in a leadership role for so long, I felt as though I was back to square one in my career. Transformation and change often feel that way. I decided to change my thinking. I acknowledged that my life and career were in transition, and I accepted the feelings that go along with that. I opened my mind to purging past baggage and unlearning, learning, and relearning many new concepts and techniques. I found that my leadership experience and executive coaching experience were great foundations upon which to build. This eased my career transition into my current role as a *Wellness Investment Strategist.* Although I felt something was missing when interacting with my clients, I knew that would come. Somewhere along the way, as I learned and applied new wellness coaching practices, I seized the movement—my mindset shifted toward feeling authentic as a wellness coach and strategist and lifelong health seeker! Controlling my thinking, actions, and feelings fueled my courage and confidence, as did the actual improvement I was achieving with my own health and wellness. I had seized the movement!

Experiencing the rapid improvement in my health status using evidence-based lifestyle medicine practices truly hit home for me. I realized I was at a point where I could still prevent the progression of chronic conditions such as heart disease, stroke, and cancer that run in my family. I didn't have to give up on my desire to live a long, disease-free life. To continue my transition, my husband and I moved back to my hometown in Pennsylvania to care for my elderly parents. My father had suffered a mild heart attack, and when I asked him if he would be open to making some lifestyle changes to potentially prevent future heart attacks, he emphatically said, "Yes!"

I had witnessed how my 96-year-old father (may he rest in peace)—a standout athlete, professional baseball player and scout, dedicated high school teacher and coach, WWII veteran, recipient of four Purple Hearts, the Bronze Star, and the French Croix de Guerre—pushed through his pain and chronic diseases every day to stay active and maintain a full life for as long as he could. I was blessed to be able to spend the last four years of his life with him, truly getting to know him and enhancing his health and wellness. I made it my mission, with the assistance of my sisters, to support him and our mother so they could both maintain their independence and quality of life using evidence-based lifestyle medicine practices. And you know what? It worked.

Sadly, many of my father's sports and war injuries and chronic disease conditions had passed the point of being reversible. However, by using lifestyle medicine practices, I was able to stabilize some of his medical conditions and decrease his medication usage. The same improvement occurred with my now 90-year-old mother—she lost almost 30 pounds, reduced her medication usage, and fended off diabetes. She remains healthy, vibrant, and spirited to this day. I've seen firsthand that, at any age, it may be possible to prevent, stabilize, and even reverse chronic diseases with the right evidence-based lifestyle changes. I learned during my lifestyle medicine certification journey that studies indicate 80 percent of all premature deaths from chronic diseases are caused by a poor lifestyle, and 1/3 of the most common cancers can be prevented with lifestyle changes.[6] It's true: we have the potential to control our health and wellness destiny through the lifestyle choices we make.

You may be prepared and ready to get started on your health and wellness journey. At the same time, it's okay if you are still a bit unsure, resistant, reluctant, or just plain scared. Changing long-standing lifestyle habits and practices generates many of these feelings, and that is *normal*. The good news is, as you complete the *Lifestyle Wellness Strategic Plan* development process, you will call upon many of the skills and abilities you already have—the skills and abilities that have helped you become the accomplished leader you are. You have been committed to being your best, doing everything you can to support your work team, *and* care for your family. Achieving your desired health and wellness will be the icing on the cake!

How do you seize the movement when you are too busy taking care of others at work and home to the detriment of making time to care for yourself? Have you noticed more aches and pains lately, are you more exhausted than before, are chronic diseases starting to set in, and does your waistline seem to be growing no matter what you do? With these things occurring, how will you continue to be your best at work and home and still take care of yourself? There are only so many hours in the day, and, as the old adage goes, *time is the great equalizer*. I know how you feel. I sometimes felt as though I was living a double life—keeping up a great act professionally in order to be an effective leader yet knowing personally I was feeling old, overweight, unhealthy, unmotivated, and lifeless at home.

How do you make time for yourself *now*? Many of my clients have said, "Yes, I know I have to *find* the time." Yes, but, who *really* "finds" the time? Instead, you change your thinking about your health and wellness and *make* the time. How do you *make time* to take care of yourself so you can continue caring for and supporting others at home and work? You stop viewing your self-care as an indulgence when time permits or something you do only after you've had a stressful day or taken care of everyone and everything else first. You think of your self-care as a discipline that you integrate into your life *every day*! You must make time for yourself *first* before everything and everyone else. Now is the time for you to seize your movement. You get to begin taking care of yourself, so you can potentially reverse, stabilize, and even stop chronic diseases from becoming your destiny. Research supports that

---

[6] Kelly and Shull, *Foundations of Lifestyle Medicine*, 18–21.

it is possible to influence the expression of your genes and boost your immunity through lifestyle changes and practicing self-care!

This evidence-based, strategic wellness planning journey will help you start your movement toward envisioning and achieving your best possible self at work and at home. Think of it as the strategic planning process for your own personal wellness. Your strategic journey begins by understanding *why* you truly want to achieve your desired health and wellness, and then you envision the person you want to be. The process guides you through what you can do to transition to a lifestyle driven by your true *Wellness Why*—one that supports your *Wellness Vision*. You create the beliefs and associated actions that work for you, so you can lead the lifestyle you envision for yourself. The time is now to stop living the same year over and over. Don't find yourself a year from now wishing you had started taking care of yourself *today*!

Throughout this book, you will see the terms *transformation*, *transition*, and *journey*. That's because the process focuses on creating *lasting* lifestyle change and resilience, and that is a lifetime journey. It is *not* a get-fit-quick program. Short-term fixes are no match for long-term problems. Lifestyle wellness requires a lifelong commitment. It's not about what you lose; it's about what you *develop*, *gain*, and *sustain*. Lifestyle transition takes effort and time; healthy behaviors must become integrated throughout your *way of life*. Becoming a lifelong health seeker requires perseverance, resilience, and commitment. These are characteristics you already possess as an effective leader. Leverage these characteristics and your innate strengths to do what it takes to become the *best* version of yourself. Get ready to meet your future self *now*!

Strategic Wellness Activities

You get to start investing in your health and wellness for the long term. The investments you make now have the potential to reverse, stabilize, and stop chronic diseases of lifestyle from becoming your destiny. Accept the challenge and seize your movement!

1. **Complete the reflective writing activity.**
   Think for a minute about why you are finally ready to take care of yourself and give yourself the gift of health and wellness. Why now?
2. **Complete the Courage & Confidence Check.**
   It's important to check in with yourself often to examine your thinking and feelings along the way. It takes courage and confidence to take the first steps to seize your wellness movement. Also, chapter readings and activities may bring up new thoughts, feelings, and concerns to work through.

WLM in Practice

Haley believed she didn't have time for her health and wellness. When we began our coaching sessions, she argued vehemently for her limitations—why she couldn't do this or never could do that or why this wouldn't work. She had built an incredibly profitable business to the detriment of her own health. She finally realized it was time to change her thinking about her health and wellness and seize her movement. Haley reorganized her workday, hired staff, and delegated responsibilities. She made time to take care of herself first and embark on her strategic wellness journey. We worked together to develop her *Lifestyle Wellness Strategic Plan*. Haley is well on her way to achieving her best self now so she can experience the health and longevity she desires in her retirement in five years and beyond.

Even my book coach and editor, Megan, seized her movement. She said she could not help but be inspired while she was completing her manuscript reviews. She immediately refocused her health and wellness efforts and began experiencing benefits within two weeks of making changes to her nutrition, movement, and work environment. She had more energy, fewer aches and stiffness in her joints, and was able to keep up with her CrossFit workouts three times per week. She involved her children in her nutritional changes and focused on creating plant-based meals and snacks they enjoyed, too.

Sheila was a busy leader at an international company. She managed people and clients across the globe, which led to her feeling as though she had to be available for work 24/7. She felt that life was passing her by. She was thankful for the support of her spouse who worked virtually and managed the children and the household. Still, the more she tried to take care of herself, the more she seemed to fail—she often let work get in the way or felt completely exhausted in the evening. Sheila chose to seize her movement only after she experienced a health scare at a work function, followed by a directive from her primary care provider.

Exploring readiness to commit can be an emotional experience. When I hit my rock bottom, I knew I was ready. Readiness is influenced by *why* you have decided to embark on your own wellness journey. You may not be truly ready; however, you may feel pressured by your doctor to make changes, or you have a desire to look a certain way, achieve a desired weight for an important event, fit into a smaller clothing size, or feel obligated to compete in an upcoming fitness event. People don't like to be forced or pressured to change by external events and desires—they prefer to change willingly. In the next chapter you will explore the true reasons *you* want to improve your health and wellness by digging deep to find your true *Wellness Why*. When you do the work, you may find that your *why* may not be what you originally thought. This has been true with many of my clients. When I work through this activity with them, it becomes quite the eye-opening experience. When you are ready, continue to the next chapter to uncover your true *Wellness Why*!

Dr. Lori's Insights

- Expect to experience uncertainty when embarking on lifestyle change. Surround yourself with people who will be there to encourage and support you and seek out like-minded friends and colleagues who share your values about health and wellness.
- Identify the people who think they are helping you by enabling unhealthy habits. Let them know that you are embarking on your health and wellness journey and provide specific ways they can support you. Those who truly love and care for you will be all in.
- Even the smallest step can have a large impact. Start where you are, use what you have, and do what you can. Don't hold back this time!

CHAPTER THREE

Why Now? Uncover Your True Wellness Why

When I think back to that emotional day in 2018, sitting in the hotel lobby feeling frustrated and out of control, I still experience those feelings as though it were yesterday. How could someone who thought she was so healthy—someone who had been a lifelong wellness seeker—be such a mess? When I was contemplating why I wanted to make a change, I remember thinking, *this can't be all there is. I can't live like this the rest of my life; I have people counting on me to take care of them. How can I care for them if I can't even take care of myself? I have longevity in my genes, so how do I want to experience aging—disease-free or medicated with chronic diseases and pain?*

Having these thoughts led me to take control of my thinking and create my true *Wellness Why*. Sure, I wanted to lose weight and improve my fitness level. I also wanted to get my lab values into the normal ranges, lower my blood pressure, lower my resting heart rate, etc.—all the typical biometrics on which doctors and healthcare professionals place such a high value, many of which can be achieved by taking medication. Does achieving these goals using medication make one healthy? Research supported that, if I made the right lifestyle changes, all of that would happen without medication.[7] These reasons really were not my *why*, but more of what would occur when I found my true

---

[7] American College of Lifestyle Medicine. "What is Lifestyle Medicine?"

Wellness Why and used it to motivate me. After a few iterations, my true *Wellness Why*—the one that elicited an emotional response for me—was:

> "To be fit, strong, and in control, living a long, vibrant, disease-free life so I can be here to care for my parents and my family and pay it forward by becoming a wellness role model and support for others."

That's a bit more compelling than simply lowering my blood pressure, normalizing my lab values, and losing 30 pounds, don't you think? Think about what makes giving yourself the gift of wellness important to you now.

Finding the true *Wellness Why* that is driving your desire for health and wellness, now and into the future, will shift your thinking and create the feelings and energy required to finally change the direction you want to go. If someone asked you today, "Why do you want to improve your health and wellness," how would you respond? Would you say:

- "My doctor said I need to lose weight."
- "My spouse wants me to be more energetic at home."
- "I don't want to have to take medications."
- "I just read an article about sitting being the new smoking."

These are good reasons; you may have similar ones. However, these reasons are extrinsic and focus on things external to you—i.e., what others want you to do or what you think you "should" do based on what you read or heard. Notice they are also all framed in a negative light.

Negative statements like these are not great long-term motivators, nor are they true *Wellness Whys*. You may be able to squash the negativity with positive thoughts, which might motivate you to initiate action, but most likely this will not sustain your actions nor increase your resilience in the long term. A true *Wellness Why* elicits visceral feelings and emotions—it's the real reason driving your desire to make changes to achieve improved health and wellness. I've had clients become quite emotional when they get there. My client Haley began to cry when she found her *why*—it really wasn't about losing weight and fitting into smaller clothes.

True *Wellness Whys* are not reasons others impose on you, things you feel you have to lose, what you think is accepted in society, or what you see in the media. True *Wellness Whys* are framed as "I desire" statements using a *positive* perspective that elicits heightened emotions. Your statements focus on things you will *gain* when you change your thinking and achieve the health and wellness you desire. Focus on what you *desire*, not what you *want*. Focusing on wanting creates more negative emotions and puts your brain into a constant state of not having. Desire is more about setting an intention or belief, which creates more "gentleness" around our perspective and is an easier place to be.

It's normal for most people to frame their initial *Wellness Why* around losing something or giving up something. This may be because mainstream thinking and research support the assertion that people are not motivated by and rarely think strategically about their health and wellness. We've been conditioned to focus on these shorter-term, tangible reasons and then fix them with quick actions such as joining a gym, taking weight loss pills, consuming shakes and supplements, and cutting carbs so that we can quickly get back to our lives as usual. Loss and deprivation-framed *Wellness Whys* may get things started but rarely motivate people to sustain health-related behaviors in the long term. Taking time to find your true *Wellness Why* will give your journey a sense of *purpose* and *meaning*. It gives you 100 percent ownership of your own health and wellness, so you can reconstruct your thoughts going forward. Who wouldn't want that? When you verbalize and visualize your true *Wellness Why*, you will experience strong positive thoughts and emotions and feelings of gratefulness that you get to take control and embrace the future you create. Your true *Wellness Why* creates a strong, lasting foundation for change—a foundation that is necessary to enhance resilience, optimism, and overall well-being.

Throughout your lifelong wellness journey, changes may occur, creating a need to adjust and enhance your true *Wellness Why*. When you are in control of your thinking, you recognize this and avoid overreacting. You take time to think through your situation and:

- Reflect on past lessons learned and what they mean to you.
- Examine the present for how improved wellness could enhance your life.
- Visualize the future contributions and the ripple effect your health and wellness could make.

To find your true *Wellness Why*, keep asking yourself, "Why?" until you find it. Your true *Wellness Why* will pull you back on track and keep you going on days you want to quit or when you encounter a struggle or challenge along your journey.

Strategic Wellness Activities

Do you have the courage to find your true *Wellness Why*? This strategic wellness activity will help you keep asking *why* until you find your true *Wellness Why*. It may take a few iterations—you will know it and feel it when you find it. When your true *Wellness Why* is big enough, you will easily find your *hows*—how to seize your movement, how to give yourself the time, and how to treat your wellness as a priority. As a leader, you may have used a technique called the 5-Whys for problem solving to reveal the underlying cause of a problem. For uncovering your true *Wellness Why*, the 5-Whys Technique is equally effective. If you are not familiar with this technique, there are several YouTube® videos available to view the technique in action for problem solving (search using the 5-whys).

1. **Create a safe space to uncover your true *Wellness Why*.**
   Set aside thirty minutes to complete this activity. Find a quiet place free from distractions. Take five deep cleansing breaths in through your nose and out through your mouth. Then rub your hands together for a few seconds to connect your creative and analytical brain areas. Close your eyes and clear your mind; stay neutral and curious. Take a few minutes to imagine what it would feel like if you had already achieved the health and wellness you desire.

2. **Complete the *Uncover Your True Wellness Why* worksheet.**
   Follow the instructions and process in the guide to find your why. Use as many iterations as you need to find it.

3. **Complete the Courage & Confidence Check.**
   It takes courage to let down your guard and emotionally go where you must go to uncover your true *Wellness Why*. The process may bring up strong thoughts, feelings, and fears that have been hidden deep inside you or that you have been avoiding. Being confident that you were able to display the courage to find your true *Wellness Why* affects your *readiness to commit* to making changes. If your *why* is not compelling enough, you may not have moved the *readiness* needle further.

If your true *Wellness Why* doesn't make you cry or create a visceral, emotional response, you may not yet be there. If your *why* is compelling enough, you will feel your readiness needle move off the chart! If you were not able to get to your true *Wellness Why*, take a break and try again tomorrow.

Keep digging deeper; you will get there. If you feel comfortable, share your true *Wellness Why* with the people who care about you and those in your support network. Also, post your true *Wellness Why* at home and work where you can see it every day. Use a Post-it® note, create a screensaver on your computer, or make it your wallpaper on your phone or mobile device. The goal is to visualize your true *Wellness Why* in your mind's eye, feel the emotions, and verbalize it repeatedly. Read it out loud for a jolt of motivation to make time for yourself and when you are struggling to make healthier choices to move forward in your wellness journey.

WLM in Practice

Nine times out of ten, my clients' initial *Wellness Whys* focus on typical external outcomes. It often takes several sessions and iterations for them to find their true *whys*. Two of my clients experienced a significant mindset shift when we worked together to find their true *Wellness Whys*. Haley's initial *Wellness Why* was, "I want to lose 30 pounds and fit into my expensive work clothes again, so I can feel good about myself." When we dug deeper, her true *Wellness Why* became, "I desire to be healthy and strong, so I feel confident I am doing everything in my power to change my health destiny and avoid another life-changing medical event. I desire to walk around every day confident and free from fear. I desire to have the health and strength to overcome new challenges and obstacles. I desire to take care of my family and am grateful I get to make things right with my family and myself."

Sheila's initial *Wellness Why* was, "My doctor said I need to reduce my stress and lose weight so I can keep my blood pressure down and lower my risk for another heart attack or even a stroke." Her true *Wellness Why* became, "I desire to be here for my husband, children, and grandchildren, watch them grow up, play with them, and enjoy having fun with them. I desire to feel better about myself so I can confidently and actively engage at work, at family events, and socially, knowing I am healthy, strong, and vibrant. I desire to be here, so my family gets to experience growing up with a healthy, engaged mother. I feel blessed every day that I get to see my family grow and thrive."

Do you *feel* the difference between where they started and ended? Stay focused on the positive future outcomes you desire. This allows you to begin the process of implanting new beliefs into your brain that overtake the old, self-limiting ones that have been holding you back. When you start intentionally thinking differently about your health and wellness future, you express possibilities versus limitations—your new life becomes a mirror to your beliefs. No more feeling guilty, self-deprecating, and beating yourself up. Your *Wellness Why* helps you think ahead of where you are.

I know the importance of uncovering and verbalizing my true *Wellness Why*—and I've had to call upon it on a few occasions to reground myself. In January 2021, almost three years from the day I experienced my wake-up call, my father passed away. My family came together to send off an incredible husband and father who greatly influenced our lives—a true patriot and American hero. His passing affected all of us deeply. My grief and the gaping hole left in my heart caused me to lose my way on my health and wellness journey.

Six months later, I was still struggling. One morning, while trying to feel productive again, I decided to organize my office. As I was reordering my wellness coach training binders and books, a folded sheet of paper fell out of my Mayo Clinic training binder. Written on that paper I found my true *Wellness Why*—to be fit, strong, and in control, living a long, vibrant, disease-free life, caring for my parents and my family, and paying it forward by becoming a wellness role model and support for others—the one I had compiled during my wellness coach training program. I think the universe was trying to get my attention! I read it out loud. I remember experiencing a deep sadness that I had lost my way, that I had lost sight of my beacon. Nothing had really changed about my *why*. I still wanted to be strong for my family, especially my mother, now more than ever. I still felt the desire to be a role model and pay it forward. I posted the paper on my office wall and decided to use my pain to fuel my purpose. On that day, I made the decision to change my thinking, re-seize my wellness movement, and live in the moment, day to day—doing what I could each day to get back on course with my health and wellness vision and mission. My father would have wanted nothing less. It took a little longer than I expected, but I made it back—better than ever. That's the power of knowing your true *Wellness Why* and letting it guide your thinking. It will pull you up when you need it, along with the people and relationships you've cultivated along the way who truly support your health and wellness journey.

You've done some necessary emotional heavy-lifting in this chapter, which can be draining. Before moving forward, take a few moments to recharge, doing an activity such as walking in nature, playing with your kids or your dog, engaging in lively conversation with your spouse or a colleague, completing a deep-breathing activity, doing a short yoga routine, etc. Find a healthy habit you enjoy that helps you recharge. Uncovering your true *Wellness Why* creates the energy for you to finally make the shift in the direction you want to go. It takes the focus off what others say you "should do" to what *you* desire for your life and desire for those you love and support. It focuses on what will give you meaning and purpose in life.

The next chapter will help you begin to embrace authenticity in your wellness journey by using your strengths. Authenticity in your wellness journey enhances courage, confidence, and readiness. At the same time, your desired health and wellness will become more important to you, and your enthusiasm will elevate to keep you believing and moving forward. When you are ready to experience the power of leveraging your strengths to support your *Wellness Authenticity*, continue to the next chapter. Let's see what you've got!

Dr. Lori's Insights

- Identifying your true *Wellness Why* is the turning point at which you can begin changing your thinking and start living life like you mean it. No excuses anymore—you come first.
- How you live every day matters and impacts those you love, serve, and protect. That's the power of your health and wellness ripple effect.
- If your true *Wellness Why* doesn't make you cry or give you that visceral feeling, it's not your *why*. Keep digging deeper to find it.

CHAPTER FOUR

You Have What It Takes— Your Wellness Authenticity

About halfway through my Mayo Clinic Wellness Coach Training Program, I again questioned my career decision. This time my questions were related to whether I believed I had the right skills and strengths to be an authentic health and wellness professional. While attending the required week-long onsite intensive at the Mayo Clinic wellness center, I interacted with other trainees who seemed more caring, more empathetic, more engaging, and more emotionally intelligent than I was. They seemed better suited to becoming wellness coaches than I did. While participating in the group activities and coaching practice sessions, I observed and tried to model others' actions, but this felt uncomfortable and even unenjoyable. At the end of day three—being the introvert I am—I was mentally drained and exhausted. Time to call my cheerleader! That evening I phoned my husband to vent. He agreed that not being true to my own strengths was not the way to go. During our conversation, I realized that, in order to overcome my feelings of incompetence and inadequacy, I had to craft my own brand and flavor of health and wellness coaching aligned with *my* strengths.

In a prior leadership role, I had completed the Clifton StrengthsFinder® assessment. My top five strengths were: Ideation, Maximizer, Responsibility, Learner, and Achiever. Strategic and Analytical were tied for number six. You can see that these strengths supported successfully achieving my wellness coach and lifestyle medicine certification goals; however, my top ten did not include Empathy, Relator, Positivity, Communication, Includer, etc.—all strengths that I thought were necessary for me to become a great coach. I asked myself, *Okay, so now what?* I was committed to becoming an effective wellness coach and strategist, so I set out to "ideate and maximize" the brand of strategic wellness coaching that felt authentic to me, in order to help my clients—leaders like you—achieve their best selves. My brand of strategic wellness for leaders and organizations fit the bill and helped me achieve the authenticity I desired. I could combine my leadership, psychology, project management, and organizational development skills and experience with my new passion for health and strategic lifestyle wellness.

Like my wellness career progression, your health and wellness efforts must *feel* authentic to *you*! Finding your true *Wellness Why* lays the foundation for your authenticity and creates the shift in your thinking and the energy needed for you to change in the direction you want to go. However, when you make life changes aligned with your true *Wellness Why*, you must feel genuinely motivated to make them. Your motivation is affected by how important making the changes are to you, your belief that you can make the changes, and how enthusiastic you are about taking the necessary steps to create the change. These are influenced by your personal *strengths* and *values*. If an action is important to you and aligned with your strengths, you will make time to do it.

From completing the strategic wellness activities in each chapter thus far, you may be confident that you have the courage to take the first steps on your wellness journey and be ready to make time for yourself. That's great—you are on your way toward building a strong wellness foundation. Even though you are more courageous, confident, and ready, you may still have doubts about how you are going to keep your health and wellness a top priority and *enjoy* it along the way. Like most people (myself included), you may have experienced several unsuccessful attempts at achieving the wellness you desire. You may have tried *guaranteed-to-work* fitness-focused programs and even diets, supplements, and medications without success. Repeated failures are guaranteed to raise doubts, make you feel stuck, and cause anyone's confidence to wane. You may now be stuck in your unhealthy "yo" like I was. You may be in the midst of your own wake-up call. It's time for you to call upon the tried and true to keep you moving forward: *your* top strengths and values.

When you are building your *Wellness Authenticity*, what strengths and values do you already have that could support this? Regardless of what you are trying to change or accomplish, you are much more likely to succeed if you identify and stay connected to the values, strengths, and abilities that have proven successful in other areas of your life. Continue building on what's already working. When you can clearly articulate your values and strengths *and* you keep them and your true *Wellness Why* in view, no matter what you are doing, you will persevere in the face of big and small challenges. What are your core strengths and values? The activities in this chapter will help you recognize the characteristics within you now—the ones you already possess that will help you be successful this time. It's a matter of leveraging these characteristics to support the lifestyle you get to have and your desire to give yourself the gift of wellness. It's never too late!

When you believe that what you are doing aligns with your strengths and values, you develop more positive thoughts, which leads to positive feelings about engaging in that activity and increases your motivation to do so. You are more likely to keep the activity at the top of your priority list. Think about an activity that motivates and engages you as a leader. This activity most likely plays to one or more of your core strengths. Do you enjoy situations in which you can be creative? Are you diligent in keeping your work commitments and achieving project metrics and deadlines? We tend to think one-dimensionally, that we only use our core strengths at work. But have you considered how playing to your strengths and values can support the achievement of the health and wellness you desire? Applying creativity and diligence will look differently when applied to your personal wellness versus when they are applied at work. You may be using your strengths outside of work but are less aware of the impact they can have on your well-being. Creativity and experimentation can make cooking more enjoyable, and diligence can be used to improve mindfulness and manage stress.

For me, I had to figure out how to tailor and apply my strengths (Ideation, Maximizer, Responsibility, Learner, and Achiever) in order to be successful and feel like an authentic wellness coach and strategist. Thus, this *Lifestyle Wellness Strategic Plan* development process was born. It pulls together the components of evidence-based best practices for wellness coaching, lifestyle medicine, mindset and behavior change, financial investment practices, and strategic planning into a comprehensive wellness investing framework to support incredible leaders as they embark on their lifestyle wellness journeys. When you step back and examine your strengths from a different perspective, you will be amazed by what you learn about yourself. Uncovering and applying your strengths and values to any activity will keep you thinking and feeling authentic, which keeps you engaged and motivated.

Strategic Wellness Activities

It's time to leverage your innate strengths and abilities. You already have what it takes to create the positive, enthusiastic perspective necessary to achieve the health and wellness you desire. At this point in your leadership career, you've most likely completed an assessment to identify your top strengths and values.

1. **Assess your current strengths and values.**
   Use the findings from a previous assessment or if you have not yet completed one or would like a refresher, try one of the suggested assessments in the guide (two are free).

2. **Complete the *Wellness Authenticity* worksheet.**

   Follow the instructions and process in the guide to identify how to leverage your strengths and values to support your health and wellness journey.

Are you beginning to experience positive thoughts and feeling a bit more enthusiastic about beginning your wellness journey? If not, no worries. This is something that takes time for everyone. You will develop strategies you can use to change your thinking and manage the doubt and negativity that often creep in. You may be remembering past failures or are viewing wellness as a punishment for living the life you have lived up to this point. If improving your health and wellness are important to you, then know this: you do have what it takes! Stick with it through the remaining chapters, and your confidence will skyrocket. Giving yourself the gift of wellness must feel authentic to *you*. As in other areas of your life, you gravitate toward what you enjoy doing. Engaging in health and wellness activities are no different. What you value or treasure is highly personal to *you*, ranges widely, and may change over time. The key is adjusting and aligning your actions with your strengths and values, and then focusing on those actions. These will be the actions you enjoy the most and feel positive about doing. If you enjoy it, you are more likely to do it and stick with it. Developing a strengths-based focus turns your perspective of health and wellness around to align with what is enjoyable and engaging.

WLM in Practice

For Sheila, two of her top strengths were Creativity and Diligence & Focus. She used these strengths every day at work. When she thought about leveraging them for her health and wellness they manifested as: "Every week, I get to use my *creativity* to cook one plant-based meal for my family that uses one new ingredient," and "When I feel stressed, I get to use my *diligence* and *focus* to rate my stress level on a scale of 1–10 and engage in a deep breathing activity until I reduce it to a rating of less than 5."

This wasn't so easy for Haley, who struggled with translating her strengths to her personal wellness. As the founder and CEO of her own consulting organization, she rarely made time for herself because she was focused on the mission of her organization and caring for her team. Her top strength/value was Fairness, Equity & Justice. She said this was important to her because, "I believe and act like every person and animal deserves to be treated fairly and have equal opportunity." As we talked through how this applied to her personal wellness, she realized she had been so concerned with the welfare of her clients and team members that she was not being fair to herself. She was denying herself the opportunity to take care of herself and achieve the health and wellness she desired—the health and wellness that would support her continued effectiveness as a leader. That was an important light-bulb-moment for her!

✦ ✦ ✦

Two of my top strengths that I described earlier are Maximizer and Ideation. I love to strategize, connect all the pieces, and create something awesome. I've used these strengths to identify creative ways I can move throughout my workday without feeling as though I'm taking time away from work or spending hours slogging at the gym. Every Sunday, I review my schedule for the week and add movement activities in between meetings and daily obligations. I don't call the activities I do "exercise" or "movement." I use reframing by making up creative names that align with my strengths and the things I value. For example, if you are old enough, you remember the 1990s and step aerobics. It was one of my favorite activities then, and it still is now. I keep my step set up in the corner of my office, always ready for a quick 10-minute *Mindset Up-Leveling*, or I stop for a 15-minute, full-body *Mindset Reset Session* or *Idea Breakthrough Session* using my WaterRower®. While rowing, I close my eyes and listen to the soothing sound of the water sloshing. I recite in my mind my guiding beliefs for my health and wellness and then visualize myself on the beach or rowing on a lake, or I let my imagination run wild, visualizing the next big idea for a future project or how to get unstuck on a current project. I'm achieving multiple goals simultaneously: mindset shifting, moving, and creating, all while using 85 percent of my muscles—no sweating required. I view my wellness activities not as *exercise* or punishment; they are quick, frequent activities to re-energize, reimagine, and refocus. They play to my strengths and what I enjoy.

Also, I work virtually, which makes it much easier to move more often. If you are thinking, *I don't work virtually, and my office is too small for exercise equipment*, there are plenty of other ways to keep your *butt out of your seat* most of the day. I've been there, too. The key is finding what fits into your workspace and your workday and reframing them as activities aligned with your strengths. This keeps them at the top of your priority list. If something is a priority, you will find a way. No need to worry about the activities and the how-to at this point. You will get there in Part 3. You get to leverage your strengths to develop specific tactics and distractions for nutrition, movement, sleep, stress management, risky substance avoidance, positivity and social connections, and structuring your home and work environments in a way that aligns with your strengths, what you enjoy, and what feels authentic for you. Distractions are used to ensure you enjoy the tactics, align them with your strengths, and divert your attention from unhealthy habits and triggers that no longer serve you. Don't underestimate the power of a good distraction.

When you begin leveraging your strengths to achieve the health and wellness you desire, especially at work, others *will* notice. You may have heard of a phenomenon called the *Three Degrees of Separation*. Some lifestyle medicine practitioners and behaviorists feel this may be relevant for health and wellness behaviors.[8] This is how it could work: your direct engagement in health and wellness

---

[8] American College of Lifestyle Medicine. "*Lifestyle Medicine Core Competencies Program.*" mod. LMC3.

activities at work may influence your work team directly (walking meetings) or indirectly (seeing you take the stairs or eat healthy snacks), which, in turn, affects their thoughts and behavior (they start taking the stairs and visiting the vending machine less often), which may indirectly influence their families and friends to engage in healthier behaviors at home, etc. Your healthy behaviors have a ripple effect—the potential to affect third–and fourth-degree connections. You have the power! What you focus on grows in more ways than you know. When you start focusing on yourself, you begin tapping into capacities you may not have known you had. You begin leveraging your strengths to create positive change in your health and wellness as well as that of others. Identifying and leveraging your strengths to build your *Wellness Authenticity* adds another important component to creating a strong foundation upon which you will continue to build your lifestyle wellness strategy. Be the health and wellness role model you've always wanted to be. Your family, friends, and work team will thank you!

In other areas of your life, you gravitate toward what you enjoy doing. Engaging in health and wellness activities should be no different. You get to be sure this time that the health and wellness activities you choose to engage in are authentic to *you*. You will feel it when they aren't—with dread, avoidance, boredom, hatred, fear, anxiety, etc. Building authenticity when it comes to your health and wellness is about playing to your strengths and values and is reflected through your thoughts, feelings, and behaviors. You *know* when you are acting in an authentic manner; it feels right, you lose track of time, and everything flows effortlessly. When you are true to yourself and are being authentic, you flex the strengths and core values you already have in you to fit your situation or role. Think about how you behave and react when you feel like an authentic leader. Now think about situations that feel forced or uncomfortable—situations where you are out of your comfort zone or situations not aligned with your strengths and values. The same is true for your health and wellness; you must find what makes your wellness journey authentic. Achieving your authentic wellness makes giving yourself the gift of wellness feel right and makes choosing health over disease effortless.

Before you move forward, if you haven't quite found your *Wellness Why*, this would be a good time to revisit the 5-Whys activity in the previous chapter. Using a home construction project analogy, think of your *Wellness Why* as the solid ground upon which you get to build your house. Your *Wellness Authenticity* is one component of the basement or slab foundation. In the next chapter, you add the second component of your foundation: building your *Wellness Presence*. I must warn you, though, that the strategic wellness activities in the next chapter may seem a bit quirky and make you feel uncomfortable. Similar to what I experienced during my wellness coach training, you might have to muster the courage and confidence to "believe it until you feel it." Hopefully you won't have to do that for too long before you begin to think differently and your *Wellness Presence* emerges. Give it a chance—it's in there!

Dr. Lori's Insights

- When you love to do something, you do it because it taps into your strengths. It's fun and engaging, and it keeps you motivated. That's what authenticity feels like. It takes time to find new health behaviors that feel this way; keep looking, experiment, be creative, and don't give up on finding ways to leverage your *Wellness Authenticity.*

- What you focus on grows. When you align all areas of your life with your strengths and focus on activities that are engaging to *you*, get ready for your confidence to skyrocket and your reach to broaden as you become a role model and exert positive influence on others.

- Everything you are doing in your life is because you want to feel something or believe you will feel something, but everything you resist doing is because you are avoiding feeling something or what you believe you will feel. Aligning your wellness activities with your strengths builds your beliefs and keeps you willingly coming back for more.

CHAPTER FIVE

Finding & Strengthening
Your Wellness Presence

Reflecting on the events of January 2018, I realized I had reached a fork in the road. Was I ready to throw in the towel on my health and wellness? Was I ready to accept and joke about my unhealthy destiny like my colleagues had? Not yet, even though my wellness cognitive dissonance had developed into a powerful force that continued to deflate my confidence. I felt I had tried everything yet remained lost and out of control—characteristics not at all becoming of a successful leader. In the past, I had always been able to overcome work, career, and life challenges. This time I felt beaten down; my confidence was at an all-time low. I was unsure if I could overcome my current health and wellness challenges; however, giving up on myself had never been an option for me. I've never been a quitter—a trait I'm sure I inherited from my father.

I was finally ready to take care of myself but lacked confidence in knowing what to do next. Whenever I had been unmotivated and wanted to quit in other areas of my career and life, I would examine my thinking and reaffirm my goals and why I wanted to achieve them, which would reignite my passion and confidence. The same is true when you struggle with your health and wellness—you must reaffirm your true *Wellness Why* and ask yourself this question: "If I'm not taking care of myself, how can I be my best self when taking care of others at home and supporting and engaging my people at work?" This is a question many people struggle with. I was struggling with it, and you may be, too. Therein lies the importance of taking time to find the *why* that is driving your desire for health and wellness.

It's difficult to be your best self and take care of and support others when you feel that your own health and wellness has hit rock bottom, like I did. I remember always putting on a good act. I suffered in silence while struggling with my dissonance, beating myself up or struggling with guilt at times. I knew I needed to make changes because the things that had worked in the past were no longer working. I had good intentions, yet never got around to figuring things out because I was letting external circumstances such as work issues or family obligations get in the way. I kept thinking and doing the same things and expecting better results. I kept fueling my wellness cognitive dissonance and digging myself deeper into a state of unhealthy frustration.

As I progressed through my health and wellness transformation, I learned how to stop beating myself up because I began to understand that I was going about it in the wrong way. I was trying to change my behaviors and actions *before* changing my own thinking. I was letting external circumstances and my past experiences control my health and wellness. I was even starting to believe that my unhealthy state might not be entirely my fault. Seriously!? I learned from my mindset coach that when you don't change your thinking first, you believe that the health challenges you face are related to external influences beyond your control. Or you may view yourself as a failure blaming things on your lack of knowledge, self-discipline, or willpower. Yes, it's difficult to resist and tune out external influences that affect your thinking, behavior, and self-perception—but that doesn't let you off the hook, nor does it mean something is wrong with you.

Change starts in your brain with changing your thinking first, but that's not what we typically do when we want to change something. We look outside ourselves, make task lists and workout schedules, restrict certain foods, and often use force and willpower to beat ourselves into submission. We buy into the belief that if we create a SMART goal and take action, use this program, don't eat this food, eat this food, take this supplement for 30 days, we will change. You may have heard that it takes 21 days to make something a habit, a myth written in a book published in the 1960s. Think about a time you put this into practice. Sure, you may have repeated something for 21 days, but did it stick in the long term? That never worked for me. If you think about it, many health and wellness challenges we face are related to what our culture and socialization suggest are normal or "good" for us—what is promoted by many business and industry cultures. The food, agribusiness, and fitness industries, sensational headlines about misleading research findings, and popular media and television commercials/infomercials shape your thinking and reinforce the merits of an unhealthy lifestyle. These include:

- Feeling obligated to work long hours
- Bringing work home and always being available
- Putting your life on hold to take care of others
- Staying "busy" all day
- Unknowingly eating foods purposely engineered to cause addiction and craving
- Eating "healthy" ultra-processed food-like items and following fad diets
- Falling for claims that eating more of one food or less of another causes weight loss
- Taking supplements to offset your unhealthy lifestyle
- Drinking alcohol to relax and unwind
- Running on lack of sleep and caffeine
- And the list goes on ...

When was the last time your boss suggested you stop working on a critical assignment due at the end of the day to take a ten-minute mindfulness break? Were you able to resist purchasing an unproven collagen drink relentlessly promoted by a popular celebrity? Did you fall prey to the advertisement about the super-concentrated fruit and vegetable supplement to boost immunity and prevent COVID infection so you never have to eat fruits and vegetables again?

These promote external fixes instead of what is truly required—a change in thinking and what we believe about our own health and wellness. You can see the challenges on the list undermine our self-care, wear us down, and reduce our confidence in our ability to ever achieve the wellness we desire. Maybe we will have time when we retire, which by then may be too late to prevent and/or reverse chronic diseases of lifestyle.

We get stuck in the cycle of putting off our own health and wellness, trying unproven tactics, and/ or thinking we are doing the right things or what is "accepted" and *still* not seeing results. We keep postponing our wellness, telling ourselves that we accept where we are, doing the same things without success, and hoping our life will be different—hoping someday we will somehow, miraculously, find more time or find that magic pill, potion, or procedure. *Hope is not an effective strategy*. Self-care and healthy habits are often viewed as a waste of time or not possible until the kids are grown, work slows down, a project is finished, the weather gets warmer, or _____ (you fill in the blank). You have hope that when you reach the milestone that is holding you back you will start taking better care of yourself. It's time to realize and accept that there will always be someone and something holding you back from taking care of yourself. I repeat, *hope is not a strategy*!

The good news is, that someone holding you back is *you* and that something is *your brain*! You have control over both using your superpower: your *Wellness Presence*. Your *Wellness Presence* includes the thoughts, feelings, actions, and perspectives that give you the poise, conviction, and enthusiasm you desire to cut through the thoughts and challenges that are holding you back from taking the first steps on your wellness journey. It helps you choose how you want to think and what you desire to believe about your own health and wellness. Your new thinking will give you the courage and confidence to begin and sustain your journey when life gets in the way—to stop using hope as your strategy. Your *Wellness Presence*, combined with your true *Wellness Why* and *Wellness Authenticity*—the strengths and values that make you feel authentic in your day-to-day activities—solidifies a strong wellness foundation upon which to build and improve your health and wellness. Thinking about your true *Wellness Why* and your *Wellness Authenticity*, what do you think your *Wellness Presence* would look like? How would you desire to *be*, and what would help you *be*? Your *Wellness Presence* is *personal to you*. It's not about what happened in the past, what you are told you are supposed to be, what you see others doing in the media, or who you are comparing yourself to at the gym or at work. Your *Wellness Presence* gives you the courage, confidence, and authority to "do you." You demonstrate to yourself that you are genuinely ready to commit and take care of you. It helps you "Be it, Do it, and Have it" no matter what is going on externally to you. Your current thinking and feeling hold you to your past, which has made you who you are today. Celebrate that and move forward. Building your *Wellness Presence* helps you do that and take agency over your brain. You create new beliefs that create new expectations. These new expectations create your new lifestyle of wellness. This is not something that happens in 30 or even 90 days. It is ongoing. Your Well-Leader Mindset™ strategic progression is always a work in progress.

Research has shown the strongest predictors of success are confidence, comfort level, and passionate enthusiasm.[9] As you can see, these manifest first in your thinking; your thoughts then influence your feelings to create new beliefs that you act on. All are components of what I have identified as your *Wellness Presence*—also known as your RICE Analysis: Readiness, Importance, Confidence and Enthusiasm. Your RICE supports your thinking about your *readiness* to make *you* the priority this time, heightens your emotions about the *importance* of achieving your desired wellness, enhances your *confidence* that you can achieve it, and fosters excitement and *enthusiasm* about embarking on your wellness journey. Choosing thoughts that foster high levels of all four of these components fuels and sustains your wellness journey. Life happens. Therefore, your *Wellness Presence* must be nurtured and reinforced by learning to adapt your thinking and taking daily actions to support that thinking.

Building your *Wellness Presence* to change your thinking takes practice. Your first step is becoming aware of your daily thoughts. It helps to write them down—our thoughts are only sentences that we repeat in our brain that are not always facts, yet we often believe them to be so. For example, saying, "I'm lazy when I get home," sounds like a fact; however, it is only a thought. You get to decide not to think this thought and choose to change it. You can acknowledge it and say, "Hello, laziness, but not today! No, I choose to be energetic instead." Then you choose to take a small action that someone

---

[9] Cuddy, *Presence*, chap 1.

energetic would do and get to be amazed at how energized you feel afterward and the outcome you achieved. When you consciously choose to acknowledge your thoughts, be okay with them, and actively change your thoughts by exerting your *Wellness Presence*, the more energetic, enthusiastic, and engaged you will be with your health and wellness every day.

You will learn how to perform this daily *Wellness Presence* building practice in the strategic wellness activities in this chapter. When you have a limiting thought that affects your feelings of readiness, importance (priority), confidence, and enthusiasm about your health and wellness, you have the power to acknowledge that the thought is not supporting you. Then take a moment to reflect on what is creating this thought, and then choose a better one. You have the power to say, "No, I don't choose that thought, I choose this one instead." This new thinking pattern, affirmation, and self-talk, combined with focused actions, will help you get past the troughs in your *Wellness Presence*. This practice may sound a bit strange, but the more you do it, the sooner you will start to think and believe that you are *that person* who gets to have the gift of wellness, and you will eventually start to feel it. Repetition and heightened emotion are the key to solidifying new beliefs about your health and wellness. That's the power of transforming to a Well-Leader Mindset™.

Visualize your *Wellness Presence* as a Venn diagram with four overlapping circles encased by your core strengths and values. The four circles of the diagram are the components of *Wellness Presence*: Readiness, Importance, Confidence, and Enthusiasm (RICE). Your true *Wellness Presence* lies within the center intersection of all four circles. This new thinking and belief pattern supports that you are truly *ready* to get started and that wellness is *important* and at the top of your priority list. You are *confident* that you know what to do this time to achieve your goals with the resources and support you get to have, and you *enthusiastically* commit and engage in creating your lifestyle of wellness while leveraging your core strengths and values. When you feel that one of the components is out of balance, such as when wellness has dropped down on your priority list due to a work or family concern, it is time to accept what you've got, examine your thoughts, reaffirm your beliefs, choose a different thought, and then get creative. Don't just stop taking care of yourself completely, which often happens. Focus on reframing the situation first; it can be framed simply as a bump in the road or a slight detour around new construction.

Tailoring and adapting your strategic wellness plan to fit the changes in your life situation keeps your self-care a priority. Your plan is never a one-size-fits-all approach. You can *always* change your thinking. There is always a better thought that would support you staying focused on your health and wellness, even under the most stressful circumstances, which is when it is essential for you to call on your plan the most. You can always find another way around or through the situation by changing your thinking and actions. Everything counts, even small actions. Your brain (your thoughts) will recognize that you are still on your wellness journey even with small actions; they don't need to be any set duration or intensity level.

Evaluate where you are for each component daily and when your situation changes. Your goal is to stay balanced or adjust your thinking and actions to shift back toward the center of the Venn diagram. Be mindful about what you experience when the thoughts you are having create imbalance in your *Wellness Presence*. Something will feel off. Changing your thoughts and taking even small actions can bring you back into balance when you are overwhelmed at work and too busy at home. Sustaining a strong *Wellness Presence* is critical for you to give yourself the gift of wellness right now and into the future, as you will inevitably face challenges that impact your life situation. Take a few moments to think about the daily challenges that have the potential to interrupt or derail your wellness journey. Are any of these self-imposed based on feelings of guilt, someone else's expectations, or your sense of duty? Other things to think about are:

- Do you put your life on hold to take care of others?
- Do you feel the need or obligation to work late at night and check email and work at home?
- Does the food industry have you unknowingly addicted to sugar, salt, and ultra-processed foods?
- Do you fall for claims about eating "healthy" processed protein foods and following fad diets?

Regardless of how you answer, these challenges mess with your thinking and undermine your self-care, reducing your confidence in your ability to ever feel healthy again. Now that you've uncovered your true *Wellness Why* and you've re-examined the strengths and values that contribute to your *Wellness Authenticity*, it is time for you to give yourself permission to take care of *you* and make *you* the priority. I know this is sometimes easier said than done. The *Wellness Presence* building activity that follows will get you started. I still practice this activity every morning and when I feel out of balance. It doesn't take long for me to choose a better thought, believe that thought, and experience the impact of the actions created by my new thought. It's your turn—the gift of wellness is yours, and you will start to experience it as well. Please participate wholeheartedly so you can begin to experience the difference in yourself. Give this activity a chance because it sets the stage for your Well-Leader Mindset™ strategic progression and your success in achieving your best self.

Strategic Wellness Activities

Developing your *Wellness Presence* helps you give yourself permission to take care of yourself first and use your new way of thinking, heightened emotions, and your strengths to build readiness, importance, confidence, and enthusiasm about your ability to achieve your wellness goals. Decide and own it!

1. **Complete the *My Wellness Presence Building* worksheet.**

   Follow the instructions and process in the guide to complete the worksheet. The worksheet consists of four activities that build upon each other to help you first change your thinking by recognizing and reframing limiting thoughts, create new thoughts/beliefs, and then act on your new thinking to enhance your readiness, importance, confidence, and enthusiasm related to your health and wellness journey. Complete the full sequence to begin building and sustaining your *Wellness Presence*.

2. **Complete the Courage & Confidence Check.**

   What are your thoughts and feelings about using your strengths to perform the activities to build your *Wellness Presence*? It sometimes takes *courage* and *confidence* to step out of your comfort zone to build your *Wellness Presence*. It may feel stupid, unnatural, or anxiety-provoking for you—resist these feelings; don't give in!

The key to building your *Wellness Presence* and finally being successful is to change your thoughts and enthusiastically see yourself as if you have already achieved the wellness you desire. What would you be thinking, feeling, saying, and doing? Of course, you know you can't become that person overnight, but you *can* start thinking and feeling like that person, telling yourself that you are that person, and doing the things that person would do. When you stay consistent, reality will catch up. Elevating your emotions and repeating the behaviors you desire will solidify your belief that you get to be that person. Acting "as if" is a great way to get on track with taking care of yourself. Be sure to make your daily actions your own and align them with your *Wellness Why* and your core strengths and values. When you do that, your daily thoughts, feelings, and actions quickly become your new way of being and eventually become second nature—a regular part of your daily routine, without feeling like you are spending more time or effort. Think of this *Wellness Presence* activity as your daily caffeine and repetitive reset for your brain—this ignites the thinking that supports your Well-Leader Mindset™ strategic progression.

WLM in Practice

Carol rated her readiness as a 4 out of 10. Her limiting thought was, "I need to wait until my daughter goes to college before I can work on my health and wellness." She said this thought came from the fact that her daughter needed additional support to overcome a learning disability, and she participated in several afterschool activities that Carol attended. I asked Carol if her limiting thought was a fact or only a thought. I reminded her that facts are written in stone and would hold up in a court of law. She paused for a moment, crinkled her expression, and then agreed that this limitation was actually a thought—a thought that was self-imposed. When asked, Carol said her daughter was not imposing this limitation on her. Carol realized she had an all-or-nothing perspective about her health and wellness. After further exploration, she chose another thought: "I do have time now. I can engage and support my daughter better when I feel better. I can and I will fit in small health and wellness actions now!" She reported she experienced excitement when she spoke this out loud.

You can see that Carol's new thought gives the control back to her; she is no longer a victim of her external circumstances or blaming her daughter. Carol's mirror phrase was, "It brings me joy to support my daughter. I get to support her and give myself permission to work on my own health and wellness today!" She chose two small actions for the week: She walked outside for five-to-ten minutes every morning at ten o'clock to reset her creativity and focus. She avoided the break room on Monday, Wednesday, and Friday by packing healthy snacks to boost her energy to finish the day. Carol continued to make time for her *Wellness Presence* reflection in the evening. Her mirror statement energized her, and the repeatable actions she chose fit easily into her workday. The energy she experienced strengthened her commitment to continue with these daily activities–her new thoughts and daily actions implant and solidify the new belief that the health and wellness she desires is possible now. Carol later decided to do more by adding a standing desk and taking five-minute stretching breaks between meetings.

Haley became very anxious when I asked her to engage in this process. She was able to choose a new thought but said she could not look at herself in the mirror and say "those things" to herself; she flat out refused! Instead, at the start of our weekly virtual coaching sessions, she agreed to review her RICE and create a new thought about her top area of concern. She changed her thought, which elicited a positive feeling, and then she was able to choose her affirmation statement and her small activity for the rest of the week. She was comfortable speaking her affirmation statement while looking at me on the screen, but not at her own reflection in the mirror. The rest of the week, she recited her statements out loud while alone and noted her feelings. Eventually, she experienced the excitement and used her mirror to show up for herself daily and own it.

Sheila was all in and very focused. Once she "got it," she used the *Wellness Presence* building practice every morning. She reported a noticeable difference in her thinking immediately. She realized that she had been using work, her home to-do list, and resentment toward her husband as reasons for not working on her own health and wellness. These, of course, were thoughts, not necessarily facts. Like most people, she was frustrated and felt powerless. She blamed people and external events that she had no or minimal control over for not achieving the health and wellness she desired. She couldn't control her husband, who was naturally thin and didn't like to exercise, and meetings scheduled at work were not always in her control. She did have a certain amount of control over her workday and full control over her home to-do list. She realized she had been using these as excuses or distractions to validate her frustration.

Sheila was also thinking in large, unrealistic time chunks versus small activities that she enjoyed integrated throughout her day. Changing and affirming her new thoughts, giving herself permission, and taking small, deliberate actions created the "aha" moment that changed Sheila's health and wellness trajectory. Over the course of three months, she was enthusiastically on her way to achieving the health and wellness she envisioned, and her husband noticed the difference and joined in to support her as well.

◆ ◆ ◆

Only you can control your own thoughts, beliefs, feelings, actions, and outcomes. You can't control other people, their thoughts, external circumstances, and events. Changing your thoughts and beliefs, however, is a process that requires awareness, repetitive action, and heightened emotion. You may believe that it's impossible for you to add something new to your already busy routine. If you are thinking in big chunks of time, then you are probably correct. Right now, it may be challenging to find an extra thirty, forty, or sixty minutes to cook a healthy meal, an hour to go to the gym, or an extra thirty minutes at night to get to sleep earlier. You fill in the blank. But what about thirty seconds or one or two minutes here or five minutes there? Think about it. Finding time for a few key actions you enjoy and then building on these actions sounds more do-able, doesn't it? If not now, when? When you create your mirror conversations, use phrases that support your new thoughts and beliefs and that resonate with you. Choose daily activities aligned with your strengths that reflect your vision of your best self. How do you want to be? Choose activities that don't require much additional effort—activities that can be done throughout the course of your day to keep wellness an important priority in your mind and boost your readiness, confidence, and enthusiasm. Your brain will start believing you mean business, that the health and wellness you desire is yours, right now.

Your true *Wellness Why*, your *Wellness Authenticity*, and your *Wellness Presence* are the three components necessary to create a strong foundation for building the best self you envision. Gaining clarity on these drives your new thought process, which will guide you to do the right things, focus on what feels right to you, and figure out how to incorporate these changes into your already busy life. Your leadership role will continue to keep you busy. Your family will always need you as well, and life challenges will be there to attempt to derail you from your wellness journey. Your only choice is to integrate a new way of thinking and believing, accompanied by positive intentions and actions, into your daily routine—actions aligned with your vision of your health and wellness and actions to help you adapt when life gets challenging.

Throughout my wellness coach transition—and even now—the two components of my *Wellness Presence* that I struggle with are confidence and enthusiasm. When I feel my confidence and enthusiasm wane, my mirror conversations on those days are about what I believe about myself as a wellness strategist and professional in the future. I do a visualization activity called a "future pull" in which I talk about myself in the future as if it were the present moment. I tell myself—or my husband—that it's time to get ready to go do my book signing, or appear on a well-known talk show, or prepare for my TED talk, etc. I quickly experience the excitement, and my courage, confidence, and enthusiasm skyrocket. It will happen for you, too. When you hit the mark with your mirror conversations, you genuinely *feel it*! You feel it by believing it is happening now and by identifying activities that leverage your core strengths to address threats and opportunities within each RICE component.

It just so happens that I am writing this chapter on my father's heavenly birthday, the first one after his passing. It's been a tough week. I've called upon my *Wellness Presence* repeatedly this week to keep me going. I think about my father's determination in his last few years, and this fuels my courage and confidence to keep going. For as long as he was able, he pushed through the pain and whatever his body threw at him. Even though I may not have completed all my scheduled wellness appointments over the past week, my new thoughts, mirror conversations, and small daily actions keep me on track and focused on my self-care. There is no need to beat myself up for missing a few wellness appointments because my life got in the way. My brain still believes I've made forward progress this week. That's the power of maintaining a balanced *Wellness Presence*.

It may not feel like it now, but you've started building a positive foundation by using the strategic wellness activities in this chapter. How long will it take you to recognize the limiting thoughts that are holding you back and that some may not be facts written in stone? How long will it take to permanently choose your new thoughts that drive your beliefs and actions to make you feel genuinely ready to give yourself the gift of wellness? Progress takes practice—you will know it when you think it, do it, and feel it. If you don't feel it, then maybe you aren't yet ready to make changes, or the changes seem unattainable. I think you are ready. You wouldn't have stuck with me this far if you weren't. Give yourself a chance and don't give up too soon. If something doesn't challenge you, it doesn't change you! Remember, it's ultimately up to you to decide how much you want to change and the duration to achieve it. Then you choose the new thoughts that drive the healthy behaviors that support your desired change and fit easily into your day. Building your *Wellness Presence* takes time. It may feel unnatural for a little while. Think back to your first leadership role. You may have felt less confident at the start, but you didn't give up. You experimented and practiced becoming a better leader every day. Don't give up on your health and wellness journey because you don't think your confidence is there yet. When you prioritize your *Wellness Presence*-building activities daily using future-focused beliefs, elevated emotions, and enjoyable actions, you can't help but keep your RICE components balanced and centered.

Congratulations for making it this far. How are you feeling right now about your preparation for your wellness journey? Like most leaders I have worked with, you are probably ready to act. Stepping back to build your *Wellness Presence* is not something you would have done in the past. A lack of courage and confidence may not be a problem for you at work. Your confidence about achieving the health and wellness you desire may already be high. Use this opportunity to validate your feelings, reaffirm your confident commitment to your wellness journey, and experiment with new, daily *Wellness Presence* mirror practices and activities.

These first chapters helped you understand the motivation driving your decision to give yourself the gift of wellness and build courage and confidence in your ability to be successful this time. Your continued commitment to keeping an open, curious mind and taking small steps toward becoming a healthier you will pay off! You're on your way to building a solid foundation that will move you one step closer to beginning your journey toward a lifetime of health and wellness, applying a series of focused, strategic, steady steps.

Keep working on using your strengths to build your *Wellness Presence* every day. Practice, practice, practice until you believe it and act authentically, courageously, and confidently. You must believe it is possible *first* because you take action based on your beliefs about the future. When this happens, you will have the courage and confidence to take the next steps in your health and wellness journey. In the next chapter, you continue your journey into a life that supports the health and wellness you desire by examining change and how to apply a constructive approach to change. Change isn't always easy! When you are ready, continue to find out how to "do change" the right way this time.

Dr. Lori's Insights

- Changing your thoughts and beliefs takes practice and more practice. Think of your thoughts as food items on a buffet table. You have a choice—you don't have to think your automatic thoughts. Move past them and choose the thoughts on the buffet that support the health and wellness you desire. Don't put things on your plate or leave things on your plate that don't support the life you envision.

- Practice differentiating between thoughts and facts. You can always change your thoughts. The past is the past. Yes, things did occur, but they do not have to define you in the present and the future. You can't change the past and don't have control over facts (like the weather, world events, and what people do or say), but you can change your thoughts about how you perceive, interpret, and respond to all of these. Respond in a way that energizes you and enhances your possibilities.

- You are human. Experiencing the full contrast of feelings and emotions is normal. Don't try to bury them or feel guilty for feeling them. Avoid reacting. Recognize and sit with your feelings, and then process them. Use your *Wellness Presence* activities to move forward when you are ready. Be sure to let others know you are processing. When you try to suppress feelings, other people can tell that something may be off. Keep doing the activities in this chapter daily to help you truly feel, believe, and act in a way that supports the health and wellness you desire.

- Break up wellness activities into small chunks throughout the day. That continuous sense of accomplishment is like *microdosing* your brain with dopamine, causing small surges of reinforcing pleasure, which increases your motivation.

CHAPTER SIX

What Do You Have to Gain?

Change happens often—and change can be hard. Did you know that nothing outside of you has to change for you to be happier, healthier, and more successful? Most of us spend much of our energy and time trying to fix the things outside of us to achieve these, but that's not how it's done. As you learned in the previous chapter, the power to change and achieve health, happiness, and success is inside of you. Your power to change lies in your ability to determine how you will think about anything, anyone, your past, and your future to create new beliefs. Life is full of ups and downs—you are not supposed to be happy all the time. Life would be boring. We would lose the contrast and richness in our lives if we didn't experience and appreciate the full range of good and bad. Like you, I could do without the bad most times; however, it is up to you to ultimately decide what you want the situation to mean in your life. Let yourself feel the feelings completely, don't try to neutralize them. If you don't like how a change or situation *feels*, accept it, and, when ready, move forward by changing your thoughts about what it means to you and how it supports your new beliefs about where you are heading. Your daily *Wellness Presence* practices help you get rid of the looping, sticky thoughts that hold you back from achieving the health and wellness you desire. When you act on your new beliefs every day you start *living* your new path forward.

When I decided to resign from my leadership role, flipping the switch was the easy part—what followed made it hard. I felt I was prepared and ready to make the change and it supported where I believed I wanted to go. I had a plan. I was working my plan every day—what could go wrong? If not for my daily *Wellness Presence* building activities, I would have thrown in the towel many times. Three times (or more) I came close to surrendering. I interviewed and almost accepted new leadership positions because my courage and confidence repeatedly waned. I still hadn't completely cleaned up my thinking. I wasn't consistently showing up every day as the successful wellness professional I believed I could be. Using my mirror conversations to activate my new thoughts and beliefs, I talked myself back into alignment. I knew I was being called to follow my passion and stay the course. Every morning, I evaluated my *Wellness Presence*. First, I practiced reframing my daily thoughts and beliefs to what a successful health and wellness professional would have. Then, I aligned my intentions and inspired actions accordingly. My mind settled in for the journey. You may not be flipping the switch by resigning from your job; however, the changes you decide to make could impact your life in a big way. As I learned, it is much easier to transition your thinking *before* you make the change. Unfortunately, sometimes you don't have the time to do so, and you end up playing catch up like I did. Using this wellness strategic planning process, you get to take time to fully transition your thinking *first*. Sometimes, with health and wellness changes, even when you change your thinking first and begin acting "as if," you might have to rip the bandage off to get started, especially when you decide to give up something enjoyable or change a comfortable, deep-rooted behavior. The strategic wellness activities in this chapter and the next will help you not only do that but also *mourn* the losses so you can finally let go and move forward for good.

I think it's safe to say you've experienced changes throughout your life: a new job, promotion, new relationship, relocation, unfavorable health diagnosis, layoff, etc. You may have struggled with some of these changes more than others. Again, it isn't only the change itself that is difficult, it's the transition after the change happens that may do you in. You can see that it almost did me in many times. I was close to going back to my past life and old thinking patterns. Making changes to improve health and wellness is no different and can be extremely challenging. If you've had concerns about your health, even scare tactics from your doctor might not have been enough to motivate you to change. You may have walked out of the doctor's office with the willpower and good intentions to change. You even thought you were motivated to make the change—but you still didn't budge, or the changes you made didn't last very long. Think about a recent change you made voluntarily or one over which you had minimal to no control. Complete this sentence: "The change I made was _____." You completed the physical act of making the change, but then reality may have set in. Thinking about that change, answer the following questions:

- Did you have to give up old habits or ways? What were they?
- Were you upset, angry, or frustrated about the change and possibly a bit resistant? What thoughts created these feelings?

- Were you unsure about how you would adapt and what the change would mean for you in the future? What created this uncertainty?
- How can you reframe your thoughts about this change? What do you want the impact of this change to mean in your life? How did the outcomes of this change move you forward?

Change isn't always easy because mindset matters ... first. Did you know that, after a change is made, your brain (thinking patterns) needs time to catch up and *transition*? If it never catches up, you could end up back where you started or even worse off. *Change is situational, but transition is psychological.*[10] Effective transition must start before the change switch is flipped. Taking time to transition your thinking before the change occurs gives you time to think through the previous questions before you actually make the change. Your goal is to be psychologically ready *before* the change occurs. When you are psychologically ready, you have constructed a new thought about what the change means for you, and you are acting on that thought to create the outcome you desire. The same is true when you make changes to improve your health and wellness. I was somewhat ready when I made my lifestyle change, but it's hard to know and plan for everything. I did my best—I believe I was 50–60 percent transitioned psychologically before I flipped the switch—still, unknowns emerged that caused me to rethink and question my decision. Staying focused on building my own *Lifestyle Wellness Strategic Plan* helped me continue to transition my thinking and practice patience. I knew I wasn't in a race with a specific end date, and I wasn't participating in a get-fit-quick 30, 60, or 90-day program. I had to commit for the long haul—for life. Not only would I be experiencing a career transition, but I would also be embarking on my own health and wellness journey. You, too, must continue to exercise patience while preparing for your wellness journey of a lifetime. At this point, you are still preparing and laying your foundation for success this time.

Completing all the strategic wellness activities will get you ready for your lifelong wellness journey. Lasting change requires you to relax, keep an open mind, stay curious, and embrace a custom approach that focuses on *you*. Transition is a process by which you unplug from the old world and plug into your new world. It begins with an ending and finishes with a beginning.[11] You *end* the same thinking and stop doing the old things first. Then you *begin* thinking and believing differently and start doing new things. The reality is that changes succeed or fail based on whether your new thinking supports you stopping what you are currently doing and starting to do things differently. You purge the old by creating new automatic thoughts and behaviors that support your desired health and wellness. Again, using the new house construction project example, effective transition requires a solid foundation. Pouring the concrete too soon before preparing a solid foundation, and building on the concrete before it is dry will affect the structure's overall integrity in the future.

---

[10] Bridges and Bridges, Managing Transitions, chap. 1.
[11] Bridges and Bridges, Managing Transitions, chap 1.

The same is true for health and wellness. You must choose, plan, and prepare your foundation before pouring your concrete and allow enough time to dry. Is your health and wellness transition foundation built upon sand or bedrock, and has your concrete dried? Uncovering your true *Wellness Why*, leveraging your *Wellness Authenticity*, and developing your *Wellness Presence* are the three foundational components to nudge your health and wellness transition forward and prime your mindset for behavior change. These create a strong foundation upon which to build.

This is a good place to ask yourself, "Am I ready to continue my health and wellness transition and begin thinking about behavior change differently?" If your answer is "Yes," continue with the strategic wellness activities in this chapter. If your answer is "No," before moving forward in this chapter, see the book resource website for a *Personal Transition Worksheet*. Complete the worksheet to advance your transition readiness—this will help you frame your transition and gain more clarity. The worksheet will help you start wrapping your mind around your readiness to give yourself the gift of wellness and initiate positive changes. The duration of your transition phase is unique to you and is based on how ready, courageous, confident, and enthusiastic you feel about changing. So don't rush through your transition. The strategic wellness activities in this chapter help you prepare your mind to begin the psychological transition that *must* occur in order for you to begin visualizing and getting ready to meet your future self.

Why do we often struggle making positive changes, even though we know we *need* and even *want* to make the change? Because we may still view changes that will have a positive impact on our lives in a negative light from the lens of our old thinking. This is often the case for changes related to improving health and wellness. The standard American diet and lifestyle are constantly at odds with health and wellness. Wellness changes are often viewed from the perspective of something you lose or give up: "Don't eat this, stop doing that, stop sitting so much, work less, etc.," versus what you get to embrace and may gain: being disease-free, having greater mobility, living pain-free, experiencing more peace, having a clear mind, etc. Sign me up! The health and wellness decisions you make every *minute* have the potential to add years to your life and life to your years. It takes less than 5 *seconds* to change your thoughts and make the healthy choice.[12] You've already been making healthy choices to develop your *Wellness Presence*. Imagine your life when healthier choices become your new default.

Take a moment to think about a change in your life that went well and one that didn't go so well. The one that went well was most likely initiated by you—you were ready and had your course of action planned out. You may have experienced a few bumps along the way; however, you stuck with it, and, for the most part, things worked out in the end. On the other hand, the change that may not have gone so well most likely happened to you unexpectedly or was imposed on you by someone or some situation, such as a surprising health diagnosis, a job loss, or a failed relationship. The change

---

[12] Robbins. *The 5 Second Rule*, chap 1.

may have happened suddenly. You didn't see it coming, and then you were left to deal with the aftermath. Things may have turned out okay, but even now you might be dealing with the aftermath.

The goal of this *Lifestyle Wellness Strategic Plan* development process is to create the conditions for the first scenario—one in which you are ready—where you identify the changes you want to make ahead of time, you've gotten your mindset right, and then you initiate the steps to make the changes happen. Your *Lifestyle Wellness Strategic Plan* helps get you ready to make the changes you desire to achieve the best possible self you envision *before* you actually make any real changes. Cleaning up your mindset and planning before you act are the keys to being better than you were yesterday, continuing along that path, and sustaining your journey into the future. At the end of the planning process, you will know what you get to do more of and less of and at what intensity level to achieve your desired self. And, more importantly, you will be able to determine if you are ready to embark on your wellness journey of a lifetime. When you've completed your plan, you might realize you are not ready—and that's okay. The most important thing is to accept where you are and start on your health and wellness journey only when you are ready. I will be here for you when you decide you are.

Strategic Wellness Activities

The wellness strategic planning process is your *time to transition*. The duration of your transition is unique to you and affected by the strength of your *Wellness Presence*—the levels of your RICE components: the readiness, importance (priority), confidence, and enthusiasm you bring to your future self. Transitioning gives you the opportunity to begin shifting your mindset and developing a clearer picture of the changes you get to make to be the best version of yourself *before* you make the changes.

1. **Complete the reflective writing activities.**
   Reflect on a time when you used a positive approach to change and focused on what you would gain; contrast this with a change that did not go so well for you.
2. **Complete the Courage & Confidence Check.**
   If you are looking for someone to change your life, look in the mirror! Only you can change your life by changing your thinking and beliefs first before your actions. What are your thoughts and feelings about knowing you may have to make some significant changes in your life to achieve the health and wellness you desire?

WLM in Practice

Sheila completed the strategic wellness activity in this chapter and reframed her change: her permanent transition to working virtually due to the pandemic. She was used to working in a large organization that supported well-being with healthy food choices, green spaces, and an onsite fitness center. After her heart attack, she engaged in her wellness throughout the day while at work, but still struggled with it at home. Her big question was: How was she supposed to work full time and stay fit without all the perks she'd enjoyed at work and without increasing her effort and time? She had already regained ten pounds within a few months and essentially stopped most of her wellness activities. She originally felt the change was a positive one but eventually found herself stuck in the past with old thinking. Working through this strategic wellness activity helped her choose a different thought. This was her opportunity to reinvent herself and engage with her family on her health and wellness journey, which was something that had been missing before. She worked on exploring how someone like that would think, feel, and act, and what outcomes the person would want to achieve. Her completed *Lifestyle Wellness Strategic Plan* provided the answers and support she desired. She learned she could live life to the fullest her way even at home!

Marnie found herself injured from working out too intensely but would not stop pushing herself. She had to lose the last few stubborn pounds, or else. She complained of having low energy in the afternoon, feeling achy, and was easily annoyed by other people. She was incredibly determined to reach her goal weight. What had started as a weight-loss program became an obsession and *fear of feeling fat*. Using the activity, the positive change she highlighted was starting and running a successful business for the past five years. She had grown her business carefully and thoughtfully. She had taken a long-term perspective about her business, but not so much for her health. She shifted her thinking about her health to act as if she was the CEO of her health and wellness *business*. How would the CEO of her personal wellness think, feel, and act, and what outcomes would she get to achieve? Her answer was: she would step back, thoroughly understand her health status and the environment, and then create a strategic plan to guide her along the way. She was all in for her wellness strategic planning.

◆ ◆ ◆

I can't say it enough: "Wellness is a journey of a lifetime." It must become your new way of thinking and your new way of life, or you will experience ongoing wellness cognitive dissonance and "yo-yo-ing." Throughout my transformation, I learned that it's never too late to make large changes or a series of smaller changes that add up to a larger change. Even though making the changes wasn't always easy, transitioning my thinking first and reframing the changes in a positive light softened the blow and allowed time for me to adapt and integrate the changes into my lifestyle. However, despite their best efforts, many people repeatedly fail to change behaviors that prevent them from living healthier and happier lives. Why do they fail? Is it:

- Not enough motivation?
- Not enough willpower?
- Not the right genes?
- Not enough energy?

Research has shown these are *not* the main reasons people fail to change. The number one reason people fail to make health and wellness changes is: most people don't know how to change![13] Ninety-nine percent of people try to fix things with action. Most health and wellness programs foster this by focusing on action and willpower: starting Monday, I will do this; I will give this up for thirty days, etc. Most programs are action-oriented and promote the *stop-doing-this-and-start doing-that* model of behavior change. This is important—eventually. However, to change your health and wellness behavior, the first thing you must do is change your *mindset* and how you view behavior change: *behavior change does not simply equal taking action*. You must change your mindset before learning and implementing new skills and behaviors. We do or don't act because of how the action makes us feel or how we think the action will make us feel—if you dread exercise, then you will avoid it, experience negativity when doing it, and will likely not continue doing it. That's why we focus on mindset change first, not to *brainwash* you to love exercise, but to open your mind to all the health and wellness possibilities that will work for you.

If you aren't ready to change your thinking or are unsure about how to change, the process of developing your *Lifestyle Wellness Strategic Plan* will help you get ready for when you are. However, you must start with mindset transition first to ensure you implement the proper evidence-based actions to create and sustain the lasting benefits you seek, regardless of how large or small the changes are. The transition time before making a change is often forgotten or rushed through. You get to give yourself time to transition first—relax and breathe through it; calm your mind and be open to all possibilities. Are you ready to start your transition and begin thinking about behavior change differently? The transition to the health and wellness you desire is all in your head, and don't believe everything you think. There is a bit more mindset work to do in the next chapter before you can begin creating a tangible vision of what you desire and believe about your health and wellness. Now is not the time to rush—it is important to take a little more time to get your mindset right about what may be changing, because you now know: Mindset Does Matter!

---

[13] Bridges and Bridges, *Managing Transitions*, chap. 3.

Dr. Lori's Insights

- It's normal to struggle with change. Accept that this is normal—don't be surprised when it occurs. Henry Ford is quoted as saying, "Whether you think you can, or you think you can't, you're right." You will struggle at times when making health and wellness changes and occasionally fall off the wagon. When that happens, go with it—don't get discouraged. Give yourself time to adapt and work through the challenges.
- When you struggle, don't give up too soon. You will risk not having the opportunity to create and design the new and improved you!
- Share with a family member, colleague, or close friend some of the changes you have planned. Talk about how they can support the changes you are considering.

CHAPTER SEVEN

What Do You Have to Lose?

It's safe to say that, up to this point, *exercising your mind* by completing the strategic wellness activities in the first few chapters has been fairly painless. At the same time, you may not think you've made much progress—but you *have*. You might not have made physical progress, but you've gained an understanding of yourself and have begun transitioning your mindset about how you think and what you believe about your health and wellness. These are both necessary to create a strong foundation for change. You've found your true *Wellness Why*—or have come close and are still in progress—and you are building your *Wellness Presence*, which enhances courage and confidence. You are aware of and mindful about leveraging your strengths and values—your *Wellness Authenticity*—and recognize the activities that align with them. You know how to approach change in a way that accentuates shifting your thoughts to refocus on what you will gain. Finally, you are aware of how allowing enough time to transition helps you prepare for change and achieve long-term success. You have a bit more work to do to ensure an effective mindset transition; however, all of this sounds like considerable progress to me—keep up the great work! I believe it's time for a quick *Wellness Presence* mirror affirmation to acknowledge your accomplishments before you move on—feel free to take a moment.

I admit that it wasn't always easy trying to quash the negative feelings and see the positive in the behavior changes I chose to make, even though evidence confirmed that my old behaviors were not aligned with the health and wellness I desired. Giving up and cutting back on wine and cheese was a struggle, and it took a while for the cravings to stop. The warehouse club cheese department experienced a significant drop in revenue as well. I never realized cheese had such an addictive power; the more I ate, the more I wanted to eat. I wasn't surprised to learn cheese contains two of the most overeaten and addictive food components in the standard American diet—saturated fat and salt. However, learning that the casein-derived, morphine-like compounds found in cheese attach to the same brain receptors that heroin and other narcotics do, was a bit of a *brain-opener* for me.[14] No wonder I was struggling to give it up—it was my go-to, feel-good food. Wine was a different story. I wasn't sure why I felt the need to have several glasses of wine every night. At first it might have been stress, but then it became a comfortable, automatic habit I never thought much about until I started to pack on the pounds—whether from excess cheese or excess wine; most likely both. Reading that alcohol by nature is neurotoxic and directly damages brain cells, especially the connections between neurons, which may be linked to decreased cognitive function and dementia,[15] gave me that extra motivation to eliminate wine as well.

Typically, when I made my life and career changes—including eliminating wine and cheese—I didn't allow much time for transition. I chose a date and then stopped. This reactive approach worked for me because I thrive in dynamic, changing environments and conditions. I always have. I would quickly embrace the change, good or bad, and remain determined to push through obstacles head-on, dig myself out, and get back on track. Without change, I thought my life felt a little flat and boring. American writer Agnes Allen developed Allen's Law, which states, "Almost anything is easier to get into than to get out of." That was the case for me sometimes. It was always easy to get into a new unhealthy habit—but it would take a while to dig out of my lifetime of unhealthy habits. I have since learned to embrace stability and *controlled change* when possible, and, most importantly, use techniques to create a positive mindset transition first. I have seen that it is much easier to manage changes when they are initiated on a positive note by changing my thinking first. This makes it easier to move through the inner struggle that sometimes occurs. Positive transition positions you for success over the long term.

You may think that achieving the health and wellness you desire will be challenging and that it will be hard to dig out of where you are. In addition, you may be concerned about sustaining the changes because you struggled in the past with similar changes. You are not alone. It may seem easier to continue making default, unhealthy choices right now, using hope as your strategy—rolling the dice, betting on your genetics, and hoping for the best—versus having the courage to make *enough* lifestyle changes to fend off chronic diseases so you can achieve the health and wellness you desire. The strategic wellness activities in this chapter will help you begin thinking about how to gently *rip*

---

[14] Barnard, "*Why is Cheese So Addictive?*"
[15] Sherzai and Sherzai, *The 30-Day Alzheimer's Solution*, part 2.

the bandage off your old self. How do you begin that positive psychological transition so you can change your thinking to create a positive vision in your mind and experience what it could be like in the shoes of the new you—you at your best self—for life? I still use the strategic wellness activities in this chapter to work through a change I am considering whenever possible, since positive transition takes time. I know if I don't make time for transition upfront, I will likely pay for it later. Not transitioning puts you at risk of reverting to old thinking and procrastination. Procrastination is an action (inaction) that comes from faulty thoughts. It keeps you focusing on the limitations holding you back, fostering self-sabotage, and creating an energy drain.

You may still believe that, even if you attempt to transition, things won't be any different this time. You've tried many other diets and programs to no avail. They may have worked in the short term, but you ended up back where you started or worse. It may seem this way because you view the healthy choices you made then—and continue to make—as *subordinate* to the default choices you make, especially the unhealthy ones. What I mean by this is: every day our culture dishes out bad choices first (*superior*), making them extra enticing, but then also tells us to make healthy choices, which may appear less enticing (*subordinate*). It's tough for an apple to compete with a gooey, cheesy pizza being stretched across the big screen. When was the last time you saw a pizza or burger commercial on television and found yourself craving an apple? Our culture has programmed us to believe *good* food includes choices with excess salt, oil, and sugar (SOS) and to eat healthily means to deprive ourselves of the good food and, instead, eat endless green salads, vegetables, and fruits. You are not wrong in thinking that sometimes it feels as though everyone and everything is conspiring against people living healthy lives.

How did your current health and wellness end up where it is now? For me, it was a gradual progression over many years. I solidly integrated unhealthy habits to help me cope with and adapt to what was going on in my home and work life. With many habits, I actually thought I was making a healthy change. My slow progression toward unwellness didn't stop until I made it stop—until I finally decided it was time to stop the insanity and give myself the gift of wellness.

You change to get into a situation and change to get out of a situation the same way—*one* step at a time. When you commit to changing your thinking in the long term, you start to notice that you make the healthy choices superior to the subordinate unhealthy choices—they become your easy default choices. They really do. Imagine what it will be like for you when it becomes harder to make the unhealthy choices instead! I'm still bombarded daily with enticing, unhealthy choices, but, over time, the unhealthy choices have lost their power over me or elicit feelings of disgust or displeasure. I know too much; I can't unlearn what I know. Working as a nurse and later studying for my lifestyle medicine board certification opened my eyes and mind to how consuming SOS detrimentally affects our body systems, internal organs, and blood vessels. Instead of the ooey, gooey cheese being stretched across the screen, I see arteries clogging, blood vessels inflaming, liver fat developing, blood thickening, blood pressure rising, and stroke risk increasing, to name a few. I now feel the need to run to the kitchen for an apple; feel free to join me!

It took three years for my authentic healthy choices to feel effortlessly superior to the unhealthy choices; the healthy options have become my default reality. *Effortlessly superior* describes the mindset shift that must occur; healthy choices automatically initiate thoughts in which you view them as your positive default options. It's time to begin thinking about your health and wellness this way by developing an awareness of your current health and wellness reality and deciding how you want to design your life in which making healthy choices becomes your default. When you get to Part 2, you will decide on the *level of health* you desire and understand the level of healthy behaviors that align with achieving it. If you are okay with the way things are, then you may not be ready to make changes. If your current reality is not acceptable—which may be why you've decided to read this book—then this chapter's strategic wellness activities will be your first step to helping you decide how far you are willing to go to create your *new* reality—to be the *new* you that you envision.

You can't change your wellness past—it's gone. You can only change your wellness present to create the wellness future you desire. You are an open book of possibilities! Once you get your mindset right, the starting point for your positive transition to giving yourself the gift of health and wellness is *not the actions* you take to achieve an outcome or end goal, such as losing weight, being more active, wearing smaller clothes, sleeping better, and/or being smoke-free. Instead, the starting point is the mindset shift that *leaves the old you behind*. Even though achieving health and wellness is about what you *gain*, not lose, you must *let go* of your old reality before any actual change can take place. If someone tells you otherwise—that you don't need to give anything up or change your thinking to achieve the health and wellness you desire—they are lying. Your current reality keeps you locked into your current default mode; it is where you are, not where you are going. You must believe ahead of where you are to move forward in your health and wellness journey—with your new thinking you get to create your new future. However, before you can begin something new, you must end what used to be. Before you can learn a new way of doing things, you must unlearn the old ways. Before you can become a different kind of person, you must let go of your old identity.

Beginnings depend on endings, and most people don't typically like endings. Habits are ingrained and serve a purpose. It's time to recognize the old habits that no longer support your health and wellness and put them to rest. They were there when you needed them, but it's now time to allow them to "rest in peace." Your current habits and routines are part of your current reality and have an impact on who you are and who you've been. Accept the fact that they supported you but must end; don't be surprised if you feel angry, sad, passionate, or adamant about giving up something that you feel has given you pleasure, comfort, relaxation, or escape. A piece of your world is being lost. On the other hand, imagine all the possibilities after you leave the old you behind and let go of a way of life you had! However, you're not leaving the old you behind completely. Feel free to bring your greatest accomplishments and the best parts of your past and old self with you. Sometimes you have more courage and confidence and feel more comfortable journeying to the future (the unknown) carrying what is best about the past (the known) with us. However, before you let go of your old identity and reality, it's important to evaluate your current reality—AKA the *old you*—decide how you feel about where you are, and then determine where you want to go.

The following strategic wellness activities help you move through the unhealthy habit *grieving process* in order to give up old habits that are no longer serving your health and wellness. You openly acknowledge what you may view as a loss. After you have changed your thinking about your unhealthy habits, the *grieving process* helps you emphatically start the positive transition process, the process by which your unhealthy habits become subordinate to your new, healthy default choices. Grieving the loss of unhealthy habits may sound a bit silly. Grieving is the natural sequence you go through when you lose someone important to you; however, it also applies when you lose something significant and give up something enjoyable. If you don't fully acknowledge your feelings, actively grieve giving up unhealthy habits as personal losses, and reach *acceptance*, you are at risk of relapse and regression to your old wellness reality. You can either let the "yo-yoing" continue or put a stop to it now, for good. This is not a one-time activity. Any time you give up an unhealthy habit or pleasurable activity, you should expect, accept, and acknowledge the signs of anger or sadness and actively use this process to grieve and move on. Keep moving yourself through the mindset transition process to become psychologically ready to step into the *new authentic you*.

Strategic Wellness Activities

You must permanently give up or reduce the frequency of unhealthy behaviors *enough* to achieve the wellness you desire—again, don't believe anyone who says otherwise. Before you flip the change switch, however, let's continue your positive mindset transition so you can manage and put to rest the associated negative thoughts and emotions. It takes time and deliberate effort to permanently make healthy lifestyle choices superior to unhealthy default habits and choices. Trust yourself and where you want to go. When you start thinking intentionally about how you get to be, you implant new subconscious, automatic beliefs and then practice believing through your actions.

1. **Complete the *Losing→Gaining Positive Transition* worksheet.**
   Follow the instructions and process in the guide to complete the worksheet. This activity helps you actively implant new, positive thoughts about what you gain by giving up or managing the habits, behaviors, thoughts, and concerns that are getting in the way of your ability to give yourself the gift of wellness now.

2. **Complete the Courage & Confidence Check.**

   Understanding how to create conditions to support a positive mindset transition before you make changes is the only way you will make wellness feel natural to you and make the healthy choice the easier choice. You must effectively accept, mourn, and let go or give up old habits, behaviors, thoughts, and concerns when you decide to begin your wellness journey.

Have fun using the losing→gaining process to support your *Wellness Presence* building and, throughout your wellness journey, to make your healthy choices superior to and more appealing than your old, default, longstanding unhealthy habits. You call upon your *Wellness Authenticity*— your strengths and values—to guide your choice of positive actions and distractions that support your *Wellness Why*. Then you integrate the mourning process into your *Wellness Presence* building when needed to lay your unhealthy habits to rest for good. Be sure to practice completing the losing→gaining process for at least one habit or behavior you've decided to retire. You might need to use this process in Part 3 when it's time to focus specifically on creating the tactics and distractions you implement to achieve your goals that align with the vision you have for your wellness.

WLM in Practice

Susan was concerned she would have to give up her daily lunch engagements with her trusted colleagues. She realized this was just a thought, not a fact—she would not have to do this; there could be another way. The group met regularly for lunch at a deli for sandwiches. The group lunch satisfied her desire for connection and positivity, which were aligned with her *Wellness Why*; however, processed deli meat, was not. Her thinking about giving up her lunches shifted to excitement about having the opportunity to become a wellness role model for her colleagues. She proposed to the group a "mindful meeting" potluck lunch two days per week outside or at another relaxing location. They would pool their lunch funds and subscribe to an organic, plant-based meals service. Susan would order the meals for weekly delivery to the office. The idea was wildly successful and created a fun, plant-based, experiential event they looked forward to. Sure, she missed her deli meat every day, so, to mourn her loss, on the non-deli days, before she left for lunch, she wrote "deli meat" on a blank sheet of paper, crumpled it up, and threw it in the trash.

Marnie was concerned she could not get past her laziness at home. She looked forward to getting home, having dinner, and then collapsing on the couch with a good book. Similar to Susan, this was just a thought, not a fact. Reading was relaxing and engaged her mind after a busy day, which aligned with her *Wellness Why*, but enjoying being a couch potato at night did not. Marnie was the leader of a learning and development department. She knew about evidence supporting the brain-body connection, which has been shown to directly impact a person's ability to receive and interpret words, sentences, paragraphs, and stories.[16] Her thinking shifted to focusing on the importance of engaging her higher-order thinking instead of rooting herself on the couch. She had been participating in a weekly book club and proposed the "brain-body" book club as their new title. The group shifted to weekly walking meetings and created a chat and voice support group using a phone app to encourage members to participate in thirty minutes of daily reading while walking at a safe pace if using a treadmill. Like any skill, it took practice and coordination to do both concurrently. The group collaboration using the phone app was all she needed to help her mourn the loss of a few days on the couch.

◆ ◆ ◆

Changing your mindset shifts control back to you to influence the trajectory of your health and wellness future. You act out your future by changing your mindset—by creating new thoughts, beliefs, and actions. Replace old recycled thoughts from your past with the new—out with the old, in with the new. You change how you feel by thinking and believing differently and acting as if—you *can* take control and give up those long-standing, mindless habits like I did. Instead of wine, I use yoga to relax and unwind. Instead of dairy cheese, I have learned to create my own plant-based, nut cheeses and bean spreads that are satisfying and healthier than the gooey stretchy cheese, although, using my Ideation and Maximizer strengths, I've learned to create gooey and stretchy too. You now get to have the opportunity to enthusiastically reinvent your health and wellness, to make it exciting and what you want it to be, and to create something that substitutes attractive virtues for attractive vices. Think of it more as a simple swap, one thing or activity for another. Your health and wellness habits and routines have contributed to who you are today. They are part of your current reality and will have an impact on who you get to become. Who do you see in the future?

You are aware now that your habits are ingrained and serve a purpose. It's important to recognize the purpose your habits *have* served for you—stress reduction, relaxation, comfort, emotional support, family or work stability, or safety. That gooey, cheesy pizza may have prevented you from starving in college or assuaged your feelings after a bad day at work. That's okay. Remember and acknowledge the past and accept that it's time to move forward, that these actions and habits no longer support the health and wellness you desire. Know that in your future lies your best possible self. Think about the habits that were there when you needed them that you must now allow to *rest in peace*. You may have to adjust the wine you drink at night, share your favorite dessert, swap out deli meat, binge-watch videos less, or be more creative about lunch and social options with colleagues. Whatever it is, it's important to acknowledge a piece of your world—one that you may have grown

---

[16] Terry, "Mind-Body Connection."

to cherish—is being swapped for a more attractive virtue, one that will support your health and wellness. Accept it. Don't be surprised if you feel strong negative emotions—even resistance, fear, and sadness—about making the change. Experiencing these feelings means you know that what you are doing no longer serves your health and wellness; they affirm you are making changes that support your desired health and wellness. So feel the normal feelings associated with transition, mourn them with positive intentions, and get ready to discover the new healthier version of you.

In the final two chapters in Part 1, you begin to shift into defining and visualizing who you desire to become—your best self. What do you believe and see for yourself along your wellness journey? You continue to build upon the three components of your strong wellness foundation— Your true *Wellness Why*, your *Wellness Authenticity*, and your *Wellness Presence*—to create a strong vision of who you see in the future. By now, I strongly suspect that you have a pretty good vision of who you see and who you get to become.

Dr. Lori's Insights

- Remember, the thought buffet is always open for business; just like your thoughts, you get to dispose of worn-out habits that no longer serve you and try fresh, new ones that will change your future.
- Cry, scream, vent, get angry. Do what you must do to *mourn*. It's the only way you will finally get it out of your system and be able to truly move forward.
- Practice building your *Wellness Presence* and integrate positive transition activities to use your thoughts to stop your emotions from hijacking your health and wellness; if you give in to your emotions, you will start the cycle of negative self-talk and feelings of failure and hopelessness.

CHAPTER EIGHT

Visualize Your Future Direction

Sitting in the hotel lobby that cold January day in 2018, I sadly realized what my baseline health and wellness was at the time, my unacceptable reality and my destiny if I were to stay on the same wellness trajectory. I didn't like it. I visualized myself standing at a fork in the road. One fork led to staying the same and the other led to making changes. Having started my career as a nurse, I knew what could be at the end of the *staying-the-same* fork: aches and pains, chronic diseases of lifestyle, medications, frequent doctor's visits, procedures, emergency department visits, hospitalizations, etc. As I watched people walk by, sadly, my thoughts were validated. I didn't have to look much further to see what continuing to live the same way in our unhealthy default world could look like for me. Then my mind's eye shifted toward looking down the *making-changes* fork; I saw a blurry vision of myself. I had no idea what taking that fork would be like and look like for me. I thought I had been doing everything I could to stay healthy and fit, yet there I was, contemplating myself wallowing and languishing in my rut of unwellness. I could visualize looking and feeling vibrant and alive, being active and participating in whatever activities I wanted, being a role model and caring for others. In that visualization I felt awake, pain-free, and grateful every morning. I had purpose and passion about life and work. I was disease-free, energetic, and engaged in my healthy lifestyle with my family. Then reality hit me like a ton of bricks. I thought I had been doing everything I was supposed to do to achieve this vision; however, the gap between where I was currently and where I wanted to go seemed quite expansive, even possibly unachievable. So why bother? This defeatist thinking shifted my mindset from the positive, desirable vision of myself to one in which my old self began arguing for my limitations, spouting all the reasons and excuses why I couldn't achieve this new vision. My arguments were quite convincing. Have you ever been there?

I left the safety of my bench in the hotel lobby to attend the next group meeting. Not surprisingly, I was a bit distracted by the negative thoughts swirling in my head. The meeting was a strategy session about how to increase client engagement and interaction with the company's technology platform. We discussed how, on the one hand, clients liked the platform and thought they were using the features properly, but, on the other hand, they often complained about the platform because they were not achieving their desired outcomes. I thought, *this sounds familiar; it sounds just like my love-hate relationship with my health and wellness.* The meeting then shifted to focusing on developing best practices with associated strategies for clients to achieve long-term success. Clients were so focused on short-term tactics and not the long-term outcomes that would lead to the value they were expecting. *Again, starting to sound familiar.* Halfway through the meeting, I experienced my lightbulb moment—I had been struggling just like our clients had by focusing on using tactics and willpower. Yes, that was it; I needed a lifestyle wellness strategy based on best practices! I saw my health and wellness efforts reflected in the current state of the client flowchart on the presentation screen—isolated, transactional, disorganized, and disconnected to tangible outcomes; basically, all over the place, grasping for whatever might work or a new, quick fix.

For the remainder of the meeting, we worked in small groups to develop associated strategies for implementing each best practice. I walked out of the meeting knowing that my *Lifestyle Wellness Strategic Plan* development process was born—or would be born soon. As a leader, I had participated in strategic planning for business development, so why not my own wellness? My wellness *is* my business. I decided to take control as the CEO and run it like one. Wellness is not something you do for a few months and then go back to your old ways. You invest in it for the long term and apply evidence-based best practices, which was the message we were trying to instill in our clients. I knew the first step in my own wellness strategic planning process would be establishing my mission and vision. This would provide the long-term focus I needed, essentially a strategy that would guide my implementation for a lifetime and be agile enough for when life got in the way—the same components as a typical business strategy! My process was gaining clarity; however, my vision of the person taking the road to change still eluded me.

In the prior chapters' strategic wellness activities, you uncovered your true *Wellness Why,* and you reviewed and solidified your *Wellness Authenticity.* Your *Wellness Authenticity* engages your core strengths and values, which defines the central *musts* and vital principles that will guide you in your day-to-day and long-range decisions about your lifestyle wellness choices. In strategic planning terms, these components comprise your high-level mission but not yet your vision. You also evaluated your *Wellness Presence*—your RICE analysis—which in some ways equates to a SWOT analysis (strengths, weakness, opportunities, threats) in a business strategic plan. Elevated and balanced levels of all RICE components ground you; they keep you moving forward, overcoming threats and challenges, and capitalizing on opportunities to enhance your wellness. These components of your *Lifestyle Wellness Strategic Plan* describe your overall, lasting formulation of why you want to embark on your wellness journey and the unique characteristics you get to nurture and call upon to be successful this time.

The last component of identifying where you get to go in the future is establishing your *Wellness Vision*. This includes your image, dreams, and beliefs for your best self. Your *Wellness Vision* paints a picture of where you see your health and wellness in the future. Where would you like to go on your health and wellness journey? How much effort are you willing to put forth to make the impact you desire? These were two essential questions I had to ask myself. That day, sitting in the lobby, I was ready to go all in. I was ready and willing to put forth maximum effort. You may not yet feel ready or willing to go full speed, and that's okay. Your readiness and willingness will ebb and flow. Throughout my wellness journey and today, when my readiness and willingness fluctuated, I revisit my true *Wellness Why* and my *Wellness Vision* to reaffirm my commitment and reel me back in. Even though you may be unhappy with your current wellness status, you may also be comfortable where you are. Understand that, when things in your life feel in order and routine, this may breed habit, making it harder for you to change. Comfort builds complacency. In contrast, chaos often breeds life and action. My life had felt in order, yet habitual and stagnant, until that day in January. I chose to embrace chaos and step out of my comfort zone to achieve the health and wellness I so desired. I knew it wasn't always going to be easy; I accepted that my RICE levels (readiness, importance, confidence, and enthusiasm) would fluctuate. That's normal with any change. I decided to focus on consistency, not perfection, because failure was not an option for me.

You are reading this book because you know you want to make changes; however, you may feel a little disorganized or unsure where to start. That's why most people jump into action quickly by making reactive New Year's resolutions that rarely stick, such as joining a gym, cutting carbs, or quitting something *cold turkey*. I read that 80 percent of New Year's resolutions have been blown two to three weeks into January.[17] Your wellness journey isn't simply crossing from one side of the street to the other. It's a journey of a lifetime that lasts a lifetime. Transforming your thinking first to change your identity takes time, and you have the rest of your life to make it happen. You can't approach your strategic lifestyle wellness with the same mindset you had last year if you want to create lasting transformation. Your outlook, attitudes, values, self-image, and way of thinking that worked in the

---

[17] Caprino, "*The Top 3 Reasons New Year's Resolutions Fail.*"

past must change before you can be open to the possibilities you get to experience in your new life now and into the future. Mark Twain said, "Habit is habit, and not to be flung out of the window by any [person], but coaxed downstairs one step at a time." Being reactive and acting quickly is not coaxing. Using willpower, force, and rigid discipline like most people use when making New Year's resolutions is not coaxing.

Coaxing looks more like this: First, recognizing the pros and cons of your old patterns and visualizing the pros and cons of new patterns to replace the old. You can then change your thinking, visualize the possibilities, and make a series of informed, evidence-based choices about where your vision takes you and your *authentic best way* to get there. Basically, you have two options: Option 1 is staying in the same mindset you had last year and going down the same path, trying haphazard solutions you hate that don't stick in the long term. Option 1 was my default pattern. I repeatedly recycled actions and programs that may have worked temporarily but hadn't stuck. Finally, I began to realize I was no longer that person, and, more importantly, my aging body no longer responded in the same way to these past actions. Option 2 is changing your thinking and choosing the strategic road to wellness—opening your mind to all possibilities and finding what works specifically for you, for the rest of your life. It's about reorienting and redefining the two options ahead of you, so you can choose the right path for you and always know that you are moving forward in your wellness journey despite the inevitable setbacks when life gets in the way. I support my clients by letting them know their wellness journeys will never be perfect—mine isn't—and that's okay and to be expected. The strategic wellness activities in this chapter help you explore your self-imposed limitations, self-doubts, and misgivings about giving yourself the gift of wellness. You get to identify the gap that exists between staying the same and making the changes to achieve the health and wellness you desire. Stay focused on *what and how you want to be different*. Resist the urge to think about what you need to do to get there. You will get to the doing in Part 3.

Strategic Wellness Activities

To move forward, you must identify the discrepancy between where you are now and where you desire to be, so you can begin to redefine and visualize your future path. I acquired this activity from my Mayo Clinic Wellness Coach Training Program. To begin, take a few minutes to visualize yourself standing at a fork in the road. You get to choose: stay the same and use hope as your health and wellness strategy or make the evidence-based changes that support adding years to your life and life to your years.

1. **Complete the *Choose Your Future Direction* worksheet.**

   Follow the instructions and process in the guide to complete the worksheet. Plan fifteen to twenty minutes of quiet, uninterrupted time to complete this activity, and use your creativity to name each fork in the road.

2. **Complete the reflective writing activity.**

   Can you commit to traveling down the road to change? Reflect on all the new possibilities coming your way.

3. **Complete the Courage & Confidence Check.**

   Choosing the road to change takes courage and confidence, both boosted by taking time to create the conditions to make a positive psychological transition before you make the change.

Think about a recent vacation or travel experience you enjoyed. You most likely had a plan and did what you could to ensure you had a positive, engaging time. Prior to embarking, you crafted a positive visualization of your adventure in your mind's eye and kept your visualization in the forefront of your thinking. The same is true for your health and wellness journey. As you imagined yourself standing at the fork, were you able to genuinely *feel it* and create a positive visual of what it would be like along the road to change? The more pros for changing and more compelling your road name, the greater your motivation to leave your default reality behind.

WLM in Practice

My clients have come up with some creative road names for the *making-changes* fork. These include: "Second Chance Street," "Disease-Free Lane," and "Endless Possibilities Avenue." Get creative and link your road names to your true *Wellness Why*. Some examples of road names clients used for the *staying-the-same* fork include: "Chronic Disease Way," "Lifeless Lane," and "Always Unwell Avenue."

Haley was focusing on creating a balanced lifestyle—building her growing business yet still having time to focus on her health and wellness to reverse chronic conditions she had developed from working long hours, excessive stress, and weight gain. She named her road to change "Balanced Barbie Way." Sheila was focused on being there for her family in the long-term and being a role model for a healthy lifestyle. She named her road to change, "Family Forever Highway." Your road names should reflect what will be in store for you when you choose to go that way.

◆ ◆ ◆

I chose the road to making changes. It is no surprise; I had many *more* pros for making changes compared to the pros for staying the same and *fewer* cons for making the change compared to cons for staying the same. I named my road to change "Energizing Lifestyle Lane," which was much more appealing than "Destined for Disease Highway." I knew I would require high energy to weather the uncertainty, sustain my motivation, and focus on changing my thinking to bring positivity into my new life and career endeavors. Which fork in the road did you decide to take? What influenced your road choice? Were you able to build your positive case for change—with more pros? What may be getting in the way of fully committing to the *making-changes* road?

This activity highlights why you may feel the *tug of war* going on inside yourself between giving yourself the gift of wellness and staying the way you are. As you read in earlier chapters, the pros for staying the same often exert a strong pull, and all the pros for making the changes may not yet be evident to you. Also, you might have noticed a large gap between where your cons for staying the same and pros for changing will lead you. This large gap could feel overwhelming or unachievable, causing you to lean more toward comfort and old thinking versus chaos, driving you to want to stay the same. One of my cons for staying the same was that I would need to take a cholesterol-lowering medication. The associated pro for changing was that evidence supported I could achieve a normal lipid panel without medication using lifestyle changes. It was difficult to believe I could accomplish this because high cholesterol *runs* in my family, and ever since college, my cholesterol has always been over 200 mg/dL. I wasn't sure giving up cheese (saturated fat) would narrow the gap.

You might have noticed a misalignment between your pros for staying the same and your core strengths and values you identified in the assessment. For example, one of the pros I listed for staying the same was that it would be easier (and more fun) to let my health and wellness simply happen to me and live *miserably* ever after. However, this was not consistent with my Maximizer and Responsibility strengths and my love for strategic planning. I strive to achieve personal excellence and transform my work into something superb. When I commit, I take psychological ownership, rarely choosing the easy route. This doesn't describe someone who would leave their wellness future simply to chance. On the one hand, you want to make the changes to support your true *Wellness Why* and achieve the health and wellness you desire, but, on the other hand, your current behaviors may be satisfying a purpose or need right now. You might not be ready because your pros for staying the same outnumber the pros for changing, and you found more cons for changing—which could be due to not being able to let go or mourn the loss of a comfortable habit. Your reluctance could be related to not taking enough time to begin your mindset transition that you worked on in the previous chapters. I get it and have been there many times. That's okay. Accept where you are—it is what it is. You will know when you are ready to move forward.

If you are feeling stuck or torn, I suggest reviewing your pros and cons for staying the same and work through them using the losing-gaining activity in the previous chapter. I used this activity to mourn my loss of wine and cheese to kick my habits. It may take time, effort, and a bit more creativity, but you *can* work through all the pros for staying the same and shift them to build your case for choosing the road to change. Stay focused on your true *Wellness Why* and wholeheartedly explore the road to change. Doing so—along with creating the conditions for a positive transition—will help you recognize and highlight additional gains you will realize from making changes, more pros for changing, more cons for staying the same, and positive behaviors and conditions aligned with your strengths that make change possible. Repeat after me: no more focusing on roadblocks and arguing for your limitations!

In the next chapter, you continue to refine your *Wellness Vision* building on the strategic wellness activities you completed in this chapter. Before moving forward, get comfortable with your output from the activities in this chapter and decide if you are ready to take the next steps in your wellness journey. Similar to the losing-gaining activity, this activity may bring unresolved feelings, negativity, and serious concerns to the forefront. To avoid experiencing these, you may have glossed over or minimized the impact of your true health and wellness future associated with choosing the road to staying the same. If you are still on the fence, the activity in the next chapter could help you get past your uncertainty and the frustration and negativity you may be feeling at this point. This might be a great point to take a short break to relax and re-energize before moving forward—before you experience the reality of who you get to be in the future.

Dr. Lori's Insights

- Have fun with the activity in this chapter. Don't let the same mindset you had last year cloud or limit your creative thinking. Transformation comes from imagining endless possibilities.
- When completing the *Choose Your Future Direction* activity, put aside how you will get there and focus on how you want to feel and how you want things to be different.
- When visualizing what is possible, stay neutral. Keep an open mind to all possibilities. Avoid letting fixed ideas and past experiences create biases or cause you to fall victim to "right" ways of thinking. Your future is unwritten; the sky's the limit!

CHAPTER NINE

The Reality of the Future You

When I hit my rock bottom, the vision of what my best life looked like was unclear to me. Having worked as a nurse and healthcare leader, maintaining my own health and wellness was important to me and influenced my behavior choices. I've since come to learn that I was not always driving in the right direction, and most times lacked valid and reliable evidence to back up my choices. What does your best life look like? It will depend on the fork you have the courage to choose and how confident you are in your ability to create and sustain a positive transition. In the previous chapter's strategic wellness activities, the list of pros you made will help you further refine your vision of your wellness journey. If you are still reading, I'm guessing you chose the road to change because you are committed to giving yourself the gift of wellness. I congratulate you for sticking with me—your commitment is admirable!

Let's say you decide to take the road to change and begin your journey. Along the way someone asks you, "When you think about living life at its best, what does that look like for you?" Take a moment. Think about how you would answer this person's question. This is a great question to ponder as you begin visualizing what it will look like on your wellness journey—and a question to revisit throughout your journey. You know your true *Wellness Why* and have identified the pros for choosing the road to change. Your list of pros is a great input into developing your *Wellness Vision*.

Your *Wellness Vision* builds upon these by further refining what living life at its best would look like and how you get to use your strengths and values to support your efforts. Your *Wellness Vision* is your compelling statement(s) or paragraph that describes you as your best self. It describes your belief about what you desire for your health and wellness and how you get to live when you're at your best. Your *Wellness Vision* may include beliefs, behaviors, actions, strengths, feelings, relationships, or a metaphor or visual image for comparison. Your *Wellness Vision* guides your thinking. It instills the courage, confidence, and energy for you to envision and live your authentic life right now.

Your *Wellness Vision* can include wellness dimensions such as physical, emotional, spiritual, career, social, intellectual, relationships, etc. When you think about yourself at your best, what activities are you involved in? Are you walking, participating in sports, cooking healthful meals, laughing with your family, or meditating before bedtime? What behaviors, characteristics, and roles are involved? Are you a parent, caretaker, volunteer, coworker, leader, mentor, or neighbor? Are you confident, energetic, relaxed, playful, focused, mindful, or grateful? Who are you engaging with and supporting? Are you playing with your children or grandchildren, walking with coworkers, participating in a group, volunteering, or supporting your spouse? These are all considerations when creating your *Wellness Vision*.

Notice that the considerations include behaviors, roles, and actions but do not yet include the *how-to*. The focus is on your thoughts, beliefs, and feelings about what your best self looks like, not how you will make it happen. Developing your *Wellness Vision* is a great time to think about significant others who will be influencing and supporting you along your wellness journey. This might be your spouse, children, friends, leader or peers at work, a coach, or a wellness strategist. Recall that behaviorists and lifestyle medicine practitioners support the assertion that healthy behaviors spread from person to person to person ... So choose your healthy support network wisely. Share your *Wellness Vision* with your network and help them understand how they can support your wellness journey. This makes it easier for the positive, healthy options to become your new default at home and work.

Your supporters may have noticed the change in your *Wellness Presence* and perhaps commented on it. Use your *Wellness Vision* to initiate wellness conversations and keep those conversations going to help you break out of old routines, mourn your losses, and develop creative and collaborative ways to realize your *Wellness Vision* today. Your health and wellness status right now is *not* about what you believed, felt, or did today. You created the health and wellness you have today from your thinking and actions yesterday and all the days past. Your *Wellness Vision* creates tomorrow's results. Nothing will change if you don't change what you believe about your health and wellness *today*.

Strategic Wellness Activities

Again, it's time to relax, get creative, and open your mind to visualizing the infinite possibilities of your best self. Use your list of pros you developed for choosing the road to wellness as an input to create your official *Wellness Vision* aligned with your *Wellness Why* and *Wellness Authenticity*—your strengths and values. Your *Wellness Vision* serves as your beacon throughout your wellness journey. Set aside fifteen minutes of quiet, uninterrupted time to complete this activity. Relax, close your eyes, take a deep breath, and picture yourself in your desired future. How do you look? What are you doing? How are you feeling? Who are you with? Take the time to fully visualize your future self.

1. **Complete the *Create Your Wellness Vision* worksheet.**
   Follow the instructions and process in the guide to complete the worksheet. Your *Wellness Vision* should feel like a stretch for you, yet attainable. Remember to focus on how you see yourself and what it feels like and looks like in your wellness future.
2. **Complete the Courage & Confidence Check.**
   Having a compelling vision of your best self enhances your well-being and increases your belief that you can and you will achieve it. Your *Wellness Vision* contributes to the motivational energy that moves you forward through the change process. It considers your best experiences, core strengths and values, and support systems to help you imagine and *believe* your way forward, to give you courage to move toward your health and wellness target while growing your confidence along the way.

WLM in Practice

I enjoy helping my clients develop their *Wellness Visions*. They get excited looking into the future and thinking about the possibilities available to them. I remind them that when they think it and believe it, they don't yet need to know how to get there. Belief precedes ability; you must believe first, that yes, it is possible, and then your brain will find ways to make your beliefs happen.

Pre-pave how you get to think, believe, and act today to experience your wellness future now. Decide ahead of time who you are and how you get to be by uncovering your true *Wellness Why* and your *Wellness Vision*. It may take multiple iterations; each iteration solidifies your new beliefs and brings more clarity to your journey.

Haley's *Wellness Vision* is: "I am healthy and strong and have the strength to overcome the challenges and obstacles of a busy work life that I enjoy. I take care of my family and have made things right with my family and myself. I am physically, emotionally, and spiritually in balance so that I am available to spend my energy on my loved ones. I engage in activities in a stimulating environment in which I experience joy and happiness and practice kindness to others and the environment."

Sheila's *Wellness Vision* is: "I am a confident and healthy person who has personal, physical, and emotional strengths to be a leader among her peers, a mentor and role model to others, a loyal friend, and a loving person who supports her family, friends, and peers through a positive 'can-do' attitude, humor, and positive feedback. I have the energy and confidence to achieve anything physical, emotional, or relational that I choose to do."

Donna's *Wellness Vision* is: "I am a loving spouse who works hard in my profession to be the best leader I can be at work. I engage with my family to provide the best environment for them emotionally, physically, and financially. I am an energetic, patient, and dedicated person who enjoys living a healthy life that incorporates exercise, eating well, and mental challenge."

Marnie's *Wellness Vision* is: "Every morning I feel grateful for another day on this earth. I have plenty of strength and stamina so that I can play energetically with my grandchildren. I am in charge of my health and feel greater well-being and contentment. I am a non-smoker for good and enjoy life to the fullest."

You will find that when you commit to creating a compelling *Wellness Vision* it will stay fairly stable along your wellness journey. I created my *Wellness Vision* four years ago:

"I review my *Wellness Vision* often to help me stay committed to becoming a healthy role model for my family, friends, and clients. I integrate wellness activities throughout my entire day, so I am not losing time away from my family and work. I include my family when possible, so we have fun together and stay engaged. I make continuous changes to my work and home environments to make healthy choices easy and effortless. I use my wellness strategic plan to keep me confident that the evidence-based choices I make every day have the potential to reverse and prevent chronic diseases of lifestyle and support longevity. I make time for self-care every day to manage my stress and wake up energetic, motivated, and ready to take on whatever the day brings."

My *Wellness Vision* hasn't changed much since then. What has changed are the strategies and tactics aligned with my strengths that I use to support my vision. Your clear *Wellness Vision* becomes your personal beacon to use along your wellness journey to guide your actions, behaviors, and the choices you make. Your organization most likely has a clear vision and mission you use to guide your day-to-day activities at work, so why not your own wellness? When faced with a choice or when contemplating an action, ask yourself: Is this aligned with my *Wellness Vision*? If your answer is no, there is no better time to refocus, get creative, and think about what you can do to tailor your action to align with your new *Wellness Vision*. Now, when someone asks, "When you think about living life at its best, what does that look like?" you have the answer—it's your *Wellness Vision*. Write it down, commit it to memory, and visualize and believe it every day. There's *always* a way to choose health and wellness.

This chapter completes Part 1. You've spent a lot of time focusing on mindset transition. Based on the remaining chapters, you can see that successfully making health and wellness changes is at least 80 percent or more related to mindset transition versus simply taking action. Anyone can act. Not everyone has the courage and confidence to get their mindset right *first*. You are the exception; you've done this through your diligent work by:

- giving yourself permission
- taking the time to take the time
- uncovering your *why*
- leveraging your strengths and values
- building authority and presence
- applying a positive mindset transition process, and
- creating a compelling vision of what is possible for you

Writing this list gives me goosebumps and feelings of excitement for you right now! I remember reaching this point in my own lifestyle wellness strategic journey. You've come a long way. It may be a great opportunity to bask in your accomplishments and share your excitement with your support network. In Part 2, you begin bringing your *Wellness Vision* to life—to your life and what feels authentic for you. First, you evaluate your current status to understand your baseline. Then you get to decide how far you are willing to go to achieve the wellness you desire. The process you will use to create the lifestyle of wellness that works for you involves balancing your expectations with *enough* evidence-based lifestyle changes that align with your expectations, which only you can decide. This is a critical concept; I suggest reading this sentence again. Balancing my expectations with *enough* evidence-based lifestyle changes ended my wellness cognitive dissonance—*forever*. Finally, I know I am doing the right things that work for me at the right level to achieve my lifelong wellness goals. And when my life situation changes, I quickly adapt. This is what *Optimizing Your Health and Wellness ROI* looks like. No more self-imposed psychological stress and "yo-yoing!" Did you hear my sigh of relief? Feel free to join me.

Dr. Lori's Insights

- *Take the time to take the time* to develop your clear *Wellness Vision*. Research has shown that creating a *Wellness Vision* boosts your positive affect and improves self-motivation and optimism about achieving the health and wellness you desire.
- Create the vision of what you truly desire, even if it seems like a stretch or too much to believe. During the goal setting process, you get to create smaller *bridge beliefs* that are cumulative and move you toward the big future vision you see.
- Positive images create positive beliefs which create positive futures. Your *Wellness Vision* is fateful. You create your future in the present!

PART TWO

The Uncertain Area in Between

W elcome to Part 2 of your *Lifestyle Wellness Strategic Plan* development journey. You've reached the gray area between preparing your positive foundation for change and actually making changes. Part 1 provided time for you to step back and focus on self-discovery and visualization to transition your mindset to believe, get ready, and expand your possibilities to achieve your desired health and wellness. You don't get what you want in life, you get what you believe and act upon. What possibilities about your health and wellness do you want to believe and act on for the rest of your life? You've learned that the power is inside of you. By managing your thinking, you create the perception you want for your experiences. External circumstances are not creating and controlling your life—the way you interpret them and construct your thoughts around them gives you the control. When life gets in the way, instead of feeling like a victim, change your thinking and ask yourself: What am I going to do with what has happened? This keeps you focused on opportunities and possibilities. Try my free mini-assessment to see where your thinking about your health and wellness tends to go. The link to the assessment is on the book resource website.

Part 2 takes you into the middle, uncertain phase of your Well-Leader Mindset™ transformation. Here, you evaluate your current wellness baseline and decide how far you would like to go to achieve your *Wellness Vision*—what your health and wellness will look like based on your goals and the balance of change and level of effort you are willing to put forth. Keep this in mind going forward: to *optimize your health and wellness ROI*, your goals, your willingness, and the evidence-based changes you decide to make must align. If you are questioning your commitment, feeling unsure or overwhelmed, or getting impatient and ready to act, then stop and take a moment to relax and use a deep breathing activity. Then, go at your own pace, but don't rush through. As before, the strategic wellness activities in the upcoming chapters are essential to your success. They build upon the previous chapters' activities and should be completed carefully and thoughtfully. Your responses are important inputs into creating a *Lifestyle Wellness Strategic Plan* you can live with. Similar to the strategic planning process in your organization, your *Lifestyle Wellness Strategic Plan* development takes time and creative thought; don't get ahead of yourself. I encourage you to leverage your strengths to stay motivated and fight the urge to jump ahead or abandon your journey altogether. Completing the readings and strategic wellness activities fully in Part 2 helps you establish more clarity around where you want to go on your wellness journey while taking your lifestyle into consideration. You identify your current wellness baseline and desired wellness goals, then examine your willingness to make changes to achieve your goals. The compilation of these ratings establishes your lifestyle wellness *Future Targets*. This process helps you prioritize your desired wellness goals and highlights what you focus on to achieve your *Wellness Vision*. Then, you structure your plan to support achieving your *Future Targets*, which typically have time horizons of at least six months or longer. No more short-term fixes that don't last. You are building your lifestyle wellness retirement strategy and beyond.

The strategic wellness activities in Part 2 integrate your levels of readiness, importance, confidence, and enthusiasm and bring another component into the mix: willingness. Willingness to invest in your health and wellness is where the rubber meets the road. What does this mean related to your health and wellness? I found many definitions, but the one that best relates to health and wellness is: "Acting or ready to act gladly; eagerly compliant; acting voluntarily or ungrudgingly."[18] Many of us are ready, confident, and enthusiastic, but we are resistant or unwilling to do enough or what it will take. This is why you spend a few chapters in the *gray area in between*. You get to run what-if scenarios to balance your goals and expectations, your willingness to invest, and your evidence-based actions within the context of your lifestyle to set authentic *Future Targets*. When you find the balance that works for you, you are optimizing your health and wellness investment. This balance supports your belief that you can and will achieve and sustain the health and wellness you desire. Get ready to gain the clarity to propel yourself toward your new life to live forever.

---

[18] Dictionary.com, "Willingness."

CHAPTER TEN

Your Current Reality

I t's time to dive deeper into your current health and wellness reality. Thus far, you've been focusing on the belief and possibilities-thinking components of giving yourself the gift of wellness. It's now time to shift to examining the physical components of health and wellness: your current health behaviors and choices. This makes up your current reality—where you are right now with living a lifestyle of health and wellness. Prior to beginning my own transition, I was enthusiastically doing the wrong things and not enough of what it would take to achieve my *Wellness Vision*. I was listening to mainstream recommendations and what was supposed to be *right*, yet my health and feelings of well-being continued to decline. I was willing but didn't know or realize what it would take until a former colleague recommended a book, *How Not To Die*, by Dr. Michael Greger, MD, that started my true journey toward long-term health and wellness. This was the lightbulb moment when I began my journey toward living evidence-based lifestyle medicine practices. My husband still reminds me of the gasps and sounds of shock and disbelief he heard from me while I was reading this book. After only two chapters, I jumped in with my eyes and *mind* wide open, which is what you get to do going forward.

However, I noticed that the book didn't focus on external things and traditional characteristics that people focus on when working on their health and wellness, such as weight, appearance, waist circumference, fitting into a smaller clothing size, looking younger, etc. I learned that these characteristics may be typical side effects when using evidence-based lifestyle medicine! As you learned in Part 1, your external circumstances do not control your life; your thinking does. Therefore, you should not let external characteristics control your health and wellness. It's time to take the focus off the external and focus on what you control. That's the next phase of your Well-Leader Mindset™ transformation. You get to see the internal toll your unhealthy life-and-death-by-chronic-disease decisions take on your body systems and decide what to do about it.

Keep in mind that *you* are always in control of the decisions you make when working through the remaining chapters and strategic wellness activities. You decide how far you are willing to invest to move from your baseline to your desired health and wellness future. I went all in, but you don't have to. My clients get to choose how much is enough and what feels personal and authentic for them. You will have the opportunity to examine the evidence and decide what feels authentic for you. Your current RICE levels may be high; you are ready, you've made your wellness a priority, you are confident, and you feel enthusiastic. You now bring your willingness into the mix. It's time to align your RICE levels, goals and targets, and willingness to invest. The more willing you are to invest by making *enough evidence-based* changes, the greater the probability your actions may reduce the development of chronic diseases of lifestyle and decrease body system impacts.

Below is my theoretical model of *chronic disease progression potential*—a red-yellow-green behavioral continuum that I am currently testing. Think about your current health behaviors. Where would you rate the percentage along the continuum? Do you think your behaviors are unhealthy, you have low control, and you tend to be less mindful about your choices (red side of the continuum)? Or do you think your behaviors are extremely healthy, you have high control, and you tend to be mindful about your choices (green side of the continuum)? Or are you somewhere in between? Next, think about your desired behaviors. Where would you like the percentage of your behaviors to be on the continuum? Would you be willing to invest in making enough evidence-based changes if you knew moving your behaviors closer toward the green side of the continuum could potentially stabilize, reverse and prevent chronic disease of lifestyle from developing?

Chronic Disease Progression Potential	Incite & Accelerate (red)			Slow (orange)		Mitigate & Arrest (yellow)			Prevent & Reverse (green)	
Rating Description:	Low Healthy Behaviors Low Control/Willingness					Extremely Healthy Behaviors High Control/Willingness				
Rating Range (%)	10	20	30	40	50	60	70	80	90	100

There are never any guarantees when it comes to your health and wellness. However, aligning your *Lifestyle Wellness Strategic Plan* with evidence-based practices and standards recommended by the American College of Lifestyle Medicine supports the belief that your actions may slow, stop, prevent, and even reverse chronic diseases of lifestyle. When you understand evidence-based lifestyle medicine practices, you build your capability to make informed decisions and tradeoffs to bring your *Wellness Vision* to life—your new reality that fits your lifestyle for life. You might be wondering what preventing, slowing the progression of, and reversing chronic diseases look like? The following chapters help you visualize what each could look like in your life. This provides the information for you to decide the investment you want to make in your wellness future. You can go all in or scale up. It's always up to you. Being the data and information lover I am, it was quite an eye-opening and motivating experience when I created my theoretical model to visualize how I could potentially impact the health of my internal body systems with my actions. This is something that I can never *unsee*. Prepare to have your eyes opened. Are you ready to meet your future self and decide what you are willing to invest to get there?

Meeting your future self involves shifting toward examining the effects your current health behaviors and choices have on your health and wellness. Your behaviors and choices affect your current self and where you are right now with living—or not living—the lifestyle of health and wellness you desire. Honest self-evaluation of your present health and wellness reality—your *Current Baseline*—is an essential step for seeing where you are on the red-yellow-green *chronic disease progression potential* continuum. If your *Current Baseline* is not acceptable, then this evaluation is the first step to identifying what you want to change. You now have an evidence-aligned theoretical model to decide how much you are willing to invest in yourself to create the new health and wellness reality you desire.

Strategic Wellness Activities

This self-evaluation provides an opportunity for you to think about where you are for each lifestyle wellness component and establish your *Current Baseline* for Nutrition, Movement, Sleep, Stress Management, Positivity & Social Connections, Risky Substance Avoidance, and Supportive Home & Work Environments. Your *Current Baseline* for each of these components is the starting point for your lifestyle wellness journey. A journey always requires a starting point. You must know where you are to get to where you envision. The roadmap you get to create for your journey is customized for your life. It's based on where you start your journey and where you see your wellness future.

1. **Complete your *Current Baseline* ratings using the *Current & Future Reality Self-Evaluation* form.**

   Follow the instructions and process in the guide to enter only your *Current Baseline* rating for each lifestyle wellness component.

2. **Complete the Courage & Confidence Check.**

It takes courage to get real and face the current state of your health and wellness with no sugar-coating and no excuses. Nobody likes giving or receiving a low rating on an evaluation. Low ratings may create discomfort, especially when you feel you have limited control to change things. That's not always the case when using lifestyle medicine practices—it's never too late to make a difference. However, the longer you wait, the more damage you may be doing to your body, creating a greater risk that your chronic diseases of lifestyle may become irreversible.

WLM in Practice

Understanding and being candid about where you are is the first step to balancing your wellness goals with your expectations and your actions. The following clients uncovered their true *Wellness Whys*, knew how to leverage their strengths to enhance their health and wellness journey, indicated high RICE levels, and developed compelling *Wellness Visions*. Their self-evaluations of their *Current Baseline* behaviors added another piece of the puzzle to inform their wellness investing decisions.

Haley was incredibly enthusiastic about improving her health and wellness. She said it took everything she had to step back and remain patient throughout the strategic wellness planning process. She was a *doer*. Her Wellness Vision included a desire to use evidence-based practices to potentially *stabilize* and *reverse* her high blood pressure and heart disease. Haley's self-evaluation revealed that her *Overall Lifestyle Wellness Current Baseline* was 35 percent. This placed her in the orange range of the continuum. Her current health behaviors were potentially *inciting* and *accelerating* the development of chronic diseases of lifestyle. Therefore, when considering evidence-based lifestyle medicine practices, she would have some decisions to make: What would be *enough* to move her toward the green range that aligned with potentially *stabilizing* and *reversing* her chronic diseases? If she developed and implemented her plan without doing enough, her outcomes would not likely achieve her expectations and could promote ongoing wellness cognitive dissonance.

Like Haley, Sheila was an intense *doer* and always on 24/7. Her *Wellness Vision* included a desire to potentially *reverse* her heart disease and reduce her stress level. Sheila's self-evaluation revealed that her *Overall Lifestyle Wellness Current Baseline* was 30 percent. This placed her in the orange range of the continuum. Her current behaviors were potentially inciting and accelerating the development of chronic diseases of lifestyle. She faced decisions similar to those of Haley. Sheila realized that changing her lifestyle to move the needle *enough* would not be a quick fix. So she decided to take more time to transition her mindset to build her belief that she could invest in her wellness for the long term.

Marjorie appeared calm and optimistic on the outside but was suffering in silence about her fears of crossing the prediabetes line. She had received a warning from her doctor and was feeling stuck—a victim of her genetics. Her *Wellness Vision* included potentially *preventing full-blown* diabetes and heart disease, which run in her family. She had no clinical symptoms at present and wasn't taking any medications; she wanted to keep it that way. Marjorie's self-evaluation revealed that her *Overall Lifestyle Wellness Current Baseline* was 55 percent. This placed her in the yellow range of the continuum. Here current behaviors may be aligned with having the potential to *slow* the progression of chronic disease development but may not be enough to *mitigate* or *stop* the disease progression as she so desired. She was highly motivated to shift to the green range of the continuum, potentially aligning her evidence-based actions with *prevention*. The key would be creating a sustainable and enjoyable plan that would easily fit her busy lifestyle.

✦ ✦ ✦

Sadly, people tend to value their health only after it is lost—after they suffer a health emergency, receive a bad diagnosis, or begin having symptoms. Getting real with your current health status helps you recognize it's time to shift your perspective. It's time to *willingly invest* in your health and *treat your health as a long-term wealth*. We work all our lives to succeed in our careers and accumulate wealth. However, while doing so, some of us work all our lives to destroy our health. That's the path I was on. I am thankful for the day I read Dr. Greger's book and had the courage to finally face my health status before it was too late. How you live every day matters—it has the potential to affect your health-span and lifespan.

It may not seem like it, but you are making life and death decisions every day when deciding what food to eat, when to go to sleep, how long you sit, whether you have that extra glass of wine, and how you choose to manage your stress. Knowing and accepting where you are is a great start. In the next chapter, you get to set your *Desired Goals* and examine your beliefs about your *Willingness to Invest* in yourself enough to achieve them. Your *Desired Goals* and your *Willingness to Invest* enough affect the extent of your *Future Targets*—what you can realistically expect to achieve. This is another piece of the puzzle to help you make informed decisions about your daily behaviors so you can choose wisely and make each day count. Lifestyle medicine has become my authentic fountain of youth and longevity. I'm sharing my journey because it might be helpful for you, too, but you'll want to make your own decisions and check with your healthcare providers before making changes.

Dr. Lori's Insights

- Healthy lifestyle practices and healthy habits are *the most important* determinants of positive health; a healthy lifestyle treats your mind and body with kindness.

- The uncomfortableness you may be feeling about the reality of your self-ratings no longer has to stay with you. You get to not let your past define your future. You always have a choice about what to do with it. Choose to be ready to put yourself first to achieve the health and wellness you desire and you believe is possible!
- Believe ahead of where you are; the people who want to stay in the current reality should get out of your way!

CHAPTER ELEVEN

How Much Will You Invest?

Y ou may be ready to go all in like I was when I experienced my wakeup call. I was ready and willing to invest, but I can say now that I didn't know what "all in" would entail or the challenges and setbacks I would experience. I created lofty goals, detailed schedules, lists, reminders, reorganized my home and work environments, etc., but didn't even come close to hitting my all-in 100 percent *Future Targets*. Instead, I achieved 60–70 percent with my healthy behaviors most of the time. Having started at a *Current Baseline* of 40 percent, technically, I was making significant progress. I kept reminding myself it wasn't a race—it was for my lifetime. I would get there. Think about your last attempt at improving your health and wellness. What went wrong? Did you experience frustration and give up after things got tough, life became challenging, or when you didn't see the results as quickly as you expected? Did you try the same thing again and expect different results? Did you resign yourself to thinking you didn't have what it takes? These thoughts and actions are common when someone embarks on a health and wellness journey. The health and fitness industries work hard to keep you stuck in a reductionist, *quick-fix-mindset* by promoting claims such as:

- This one diet is the best!
- This exercise program will burn belly fat!

- Eat this one food to lose weight!
- Use this supplement to improve your memory!
- Use this protein powder to build muscle without lifting weights!
- Take this supplement to fall asleep fast!

Why is it so easy to fall back into or stay in a fixed-mindset focused on *fast* results when it comes to our health and wellness? It may be that you haven't developed the strong foundation for exercising a growth mindset—an important component of your Well-Leader Mindset™ strategic progression—when it comes to changing your health and wellness. The claims in the list are just that, claims or thoughts provided by others, not necessarily evidence based. An important characteristic of a growth mindset is being able to discern evidence-based practices from unsupported thoughts or claims. The process of developing your *Lifestyle Wellness Strategic Plan* will help you do this. Developing a growth mindset is critical to giving yourself the gift of wellness and reaching higher levels of achievement this time. Without a strategic perspective and a growth mindset, there is a strong probability you won't do enough of what it will take or you may hurt yourself by doing too much. You could remain stuck in your old ways and miss out on the evidence-based, collaborative opportunities available to support your wellness journey.

What is a growth mindset, and why is it essential to achieving your desired health and wellness? Growth mindsets allow you to be open to learning new things to improve health and wellness and question old beliefs and quick-fix programs that may not be working or haven't worked in the past. Those with growth mindsets experiment with new techniques that require stepping out of your comfort zone to improve skills and capabilities. They embrace change and persist in the face of setbacks and challenges. Instead of feeling frustrated and giving up when challenges arise, people with growth mindsets think creatively to adapt and integrate new programs and activities to keep moving forward. They recognize they will make mistakes, and failures will occur. These are a normal part of growth, provide new information for more action, and support learning and self-discovery. They welcome feedback and find lessons and inspiration from others. Not all health and wellness activities are going to work. Frequent evaluation, discussion, and feedback help people with growth mindsets learn and experiment with different techniques to continue to grow.

You may feel you exhibit a growth mindset in other areas of your life. However, there is something extremely personal about health and wellness that makes people easily shift into a defensive, "I've-Tried-It-All," or "I-Know-What-To-Do" fixed-mindset mode. This thinking closes our minds to personalized, evidence-based lifestyle changes that could add years to our lives and life to our years. Mindsets are self-fulfilling prophecies—if you think you can improve, you will. If you think you are stuck, you are. The good news is that mindsets are learned and can be transformed by changing our thoughts and deciding what we get to do with the situations we experience. A growth mindset thrives on challenge and sees failure not as evidence of incompetence or unintelligence but as a springboard for learning and more growth. Overcoming challenges stretches your existing abilities and elevates all possibilities available to you.

Achieving your *Wellness Vision* is possible when you commit to a growth mindset when developing your authentic *Lifestyle Wellness Strategic Plan*. When you are ready to implement your plan, you get to experiment with new ideas and embrace both your successes and "less than successes" (no such thing as failures here). You never fail; you learn, adapt, and move forward. French philosopher Henri Bergson once said, "To exist is to change, to change is to mature; to mature is to go on creating oneself endlessly." Your wellness journey should foster a spirit of entrepreneurship and willingness to invest in yourself and step out of your comfort zone by trying new evidence-based methods to achieve your wellness goals. A growth mindset opens your eyes so you get to view your health and wellness journey through the lens of new possibilities.

In this chapter's strategic wellness activities, you get to add the remaining pieces of your self-evaluation: your *Desired Goal* and *Willingness to Invest* ratings. These, combined with your *Current Baseline*, form your composite *Future Target* for each lifestyle wellness component and your *Overall Lifestyle Wellness Future Target*. As you did with your *Current Baseline* ratings, provide candid, thoughtful ratings to ensure your initial *Future Targets* reflect the overall lifestyle wellness you seek. For now, you are merely choosing a starting point; you get to adjust your targets as needed until they feel authentic and achievable. Your *Future Target* for each lifestyle wellness component reflects your authentic (red-yellow-green) future state that will support and sustain your *Wellness Vision*. The higher your *Future Targets*, the more possibilities await outside your comfort zone. The more you step out of your comfort zone, the greater probability your evidence-based behaviors have the potential to slow, mitigate, prevent, and even reverse chronic diseases of lifestyle.

How much are you willing to invest? When it's time to set your *Future Targets*, you may decide you are only willing to make enough changes to move into the light orange-yellow range of the continuum, which increases the probability that your actions may slow the progression of chronic diseases of lifestyle. However, this may not be enough, and your healthcare provider may suggest you begin taking or continue taking medications. On the other hand, making a few more changes to move into the green area of the continuum may increase the probability that your actions could mitigate and stop the progression of chronic diseases and possibly eliminate the need for medication. You get to decide. Research supports that making changes in every lifestyle wellness component has the potential to affect the health and functioning of all body systems (e.g., cardiovascular, respiratory, digestive, urinary, immune, etc.), including strengthening immune function, reducing inflammation in your heart and blood vessels, reducing your cancer risk, and boosting mood and memory. The choice is always yours; however, always consult with your healthcare provider before making any health and wellness changes that could impact existing health conditions and medication usage. This time, you get to make informed choices and tradeoffs versus simply hoping for the best.

Strategic Wellness Activities

In the previous chapter's strategic wellness activities, you identified your *Current Baseline* ratings for each lifestyle wellness component. It's now time to think about what you want your future to look like—how you want your *Wellness Vision* to play out. Believe ahead of where you are; your thoughts create your future.

1. **Add your *Desired Goal* and *Willingness to Invest* ratings.**
   Use the *Current & Future Reality Self-Evaluation* form from the previous chapter's strategic wellness activities. Follow the instructions and process in the guide to enter your ratings for each lifestyle wellness component. The form will calculate your initial *Future Target* and *Overall Lifestyle Wellness* ratings.
2. **Conduct a final review of all your self-ratings.**
   Review your self-ratings to ensure you are satisfied with them and that they reflect your current self and desired future self.
3. **Complete the Courage & Confidence Check.**
   Your courage and confidence may impact your willingness to invest in your health and wellness future. You're open to keeping a growth mindset, you've identified your baseline for each component, and you've chosen your goal, yet you still may feel hesitant or unsure about your ability to pull it off. It's normal that you may feel a bit unwilling to make changes. Willingness to invest is enhanced by being prepared—you are not yet fully prepared. As you complete additional sections of your *Lifestyle Wellness Strategic Plan*, your path to the health and wellness you desire becomes more tangible, believable, and doable in your mind. As a result, your confidence and courage build; you can, and you will be prepared to take the next steps on your journey. Keep moving forward.

If you feel unsure about your self-evaluation, no worries—your goals and targets are not carved in stone. You get to adjust them when developing your tactics and distractions to achieve each target. Then, you will have a better idea about whether or not you can realistically achieve the goals and targets you've set within the context of your busy life; you may decide to start smaller or realize you are ready to play big! Your focus is on making your goals and targets feel authentic to you and what fits your lifestyle. Don't let your fear of change get in the way. Fear of making a change is normal. Then again, how long do you want to stay in your current reality? Imagine what life would be like if you didn't; stop imagining and start experiencing!

Tempering your *Desired Goals* and *Future Targets* with your *Willingness to Invest* and the likelihood you can make enough changes is the key to creating an authentic *Lifestyle Wellness Strategic*

Plan you can and will live with. The following client examples build upon those in the previous chapters. They illustrate how clients apply an iterative process to resolve their wellness cognitive dissonance and ensure they authentically live their *Wellness Visions* by aligning their thoughts, beliefs, and actions.

WLM in Practice

Haley's *Wellness Vision* included a desire to *reverse* her high blood pressure and heart disease. Her *Overall Lifestyle Wellness Current Baseline* average was 35 percent. Her *Desired Goal* was 90 percent; however, based on her *Willingness to Invest* ratings and what she felt she could likely achieve, her *Overall Lifestyle Wellness Future Target* calculated to 60 percent. This target was in the yellow range of the continuum aligned with the possibility that her actions at this level could potentially *mitigate* and *arrest* her current chronic diseases of lifestyle. She decided this was a great place to start and committed to achieving 60 percent over the next year. Haley chose the *authentic* level she believed she could invest in and consistently fit into her current work-life demands—belief before action.

Sheila's commitment was similar to Haley's. Her *Wellness Vision* included a desire to *reverse* her heart disease and manage stress. Her *Overall Desired Goal* was 100 percent, which was supported by her *Willingness to Invest* and *Future Targets*. However, her *Overall Lifestyle Wellness Current Baseline* was only 30 percent, located in the red-orange range of the continuum. This location aligned with her actions potentially continuing to incite her chronic disease development. Even though her *Willingness to Invest* was 100 percent, realistically, moving from 30 to 100 percent presented a significant gap to close. She knew the likelihood she could go all in was much lower. She had used this all-in approach without success; her efforts lasted about three weeks. Sheila decided to focus on changing her mindset. She knew that when she got to the detailed planning process, she would start with smaller steps she could build upon to achieve her *Future Targets*. Sheila reprogramed her thinking and beliefs to see herself achieving smaller incremental changes over a longer duration. She used her *Wellness Presence* building and positive transition activities to solidify her belief that slow and steady was a great way to start. She felt blessed to get this opportunity to move her health and wellness to the top of her priority list.

Marjorie's *Wellness Vision* included a desire to *prevent* diabetes and heart disease, which run in her family. Her *Overall Lifestyle Wellness Current Baseline* was 55 percent. She was asymptomatic and not taking medication. Her *Desired Goal* was 100 percent; however, based on her *Willingness to Invest* and what she felt likely to achieve, her *Overall Lifestyle Wellness Future Target* was 75 percent. This target is in the light-green range of the continuum, aligned with her actions potentially mitigating and arresting chronic disease development. It may not be quite enough to potentially prevent them.

The change that would move Marjorie's needle the most was related to her nutrition. It is important to note here that when it comes to food choices, preventing chronic diseases from occurring when a person is still disease-free may require less effort than when already starting to experience symptoms.[19] Marjorie's motivation and willingness were high, and the good news for her was that she could potentially stabilize her disease progression by starting with fewer changes. Her plan could allow for flexibility and sustainability by starting at 75 percent, experimenting with what would work best for her, and progressing when she felt ready.

◆ ◆ ◆

As with any journey or adventure (or vacation), preparation is the key. When I began my health and wellness journey, I was unprepared—courageous and willing, but unprepared. Even though I was committed to staying the course, I experienced many challenges due to being unprepared and reactive. That's why I created this *Lifestyle Wellness Strategic Plan* development process—to help you take time to get prepared and ready for your wellness journey of a lifetime. I'm also a certified Project Management Professional (PMP®) through the Project Management Institute (PMI). I've learned that a best practice for planning a long-duration project is to avoid extending your planning horizon too far into the future—it's best to use three-to-six-month interim horizons. Also, when it comes to planning, it's impossible to develop a contingency plan for everything. When you begin your detailed planning, you may decide to shift your goals and targets to align with shorter planning horizons. Also, the resilience and sustainment tactics you devise will support continued mindset transition by dimming limitations, managing your thinking, and solidifying your beliefs to keep you focused on growth and endless possibilities. When you stay focused on *growth* as your outcome, your perspective changes—you view challenges as opportunities to call upon your strengths and flex your creativity and problem-solving abilities to create new possibilities.

You've completed all the foundational inputs and get to take your plan to the next level of detail. You've identified your starting point, why you want to go there, what strengths and support you have available to leverage, where you want to go, what it looks like, and what you want to achieve when you get there. However, your tactics, distractions, and logistics are still to come as well as tactics to keep you motivated and moving forward when life happens. You will work on these in Part 3. It's time to organize and document your plan. In the next chapter's strategic wellness activities, you take time to review your work thus far and enter key inputs into the *Lifestyle Wellness Strategic Plan Template*. You will see that your plan is starting to come together into one cohesive document to support achieving your desired health and wellness. You will complete all components of your *Lifestyle*

---

[19] Campbell, "*How Strict Does My Plant-Based Diet Need To Be?*"

Wellness Strategic Plan by the end of this book. Your custom plan will be ready to implement when you start your authentic journey to optimize your health and wellness investment.

A growth and possibilities mindset is critical to giving yourself the gift of wellness and potentially stabilizing, preventing, and reversing the progression of chronic diseases of lifestyle. How far are you willing to go now, and will this be *enough* to support your *Wellness Why* and experience your *Wellness Vision*? Your *Lifestyle Wellness Strategic Plan* development process provides the answers to these questions. You can always do more or scale back to achieve authenticity. When you choose your tactics and distractions, you can adjust your *Future Targets* as needed. Changing and adapting are normal when developing a plan and ongoing after you implement your plan. There is a huge difference between saying, "I am not ready for this" and "I am not ready for this *yet*." Adding *yet* suggests you will get there with more practice and perseverance. Embracing a growth mindset and fully engaging in creating your *Lifestyle Wellness Strategic Plan* begins the process of getting unstuck from your old ways and increasing your Willingness to Invest in You!

Dr. Lori's Insights

- When it comes to your health, don't rush to "I can't" when faced with making a change to an ingrained habit. With a bit of creativity, you might surprise yourself by how easy it is to make the change *and* you might actually enjoy it.
- Your body is the *only one* you have. If you envision yourself enjoying an active, disease-free, and medication-free lifestyle, you are on your way to breaking the cycle of wellness failure. You've learned that it takes a planned, strategic approach to make this happen. You may not think you are good at strategizing and planning, but that's just a thought, not a fact. Adding yet to the end of that sentence sets your future belief in your new ability; your quality of life and longevity depend on it!
- Embracing a growth mindset to achieve your desired health and wellness takes commitment, time, and patience. In addition, it takes a strategic perspective and an iterative, evidence-based approach to envision what *authenticity* looks like for your busy lifestyle.

CHAPTER TWELVE

Your Lifestyle Wellness Strategic Plan

After five years, I finally see myself as the CEO of my own health and wellness destiny; it's my second "business." I run it using my own *Lifestyle Wellness Strategic Plan*. I'm confident that completing the strategic wellness activities thus far has inspired you to begin thinking about your health and wellness from an entrepreneurial, growth-mindset perspective. It's time for you to *invest* in your new beginning. It's time for a release of energy in a new direction toward achieving your best self. Your *Lifestyle Wellness Strategic Plan* supports your authentic journey to optimize your health and wellness. This is a great point to step back, reflect, and begin compiling your plan using the *LWSP template* found on the book resource website. The guide contains more detailed instructions and tips to help you compile your plan. You will see how all the pieces fit together to support your Well-Leader Mindset™ strategic progression.

Your *Lifestyle Wellness Strategic Plan* contains ten sections. You've completed the inputs for the first four sections:

1.0: My Wellness Mission, Vision, & Aspirations
2.0: My Wellness Authenticity
3.0: My Wellness Presence—RICE Analysis
4.0: My Lifestyle Wellness Investment Goals & Targets

These four sections support your mindset shift and elevate your courage and confidence to commit to giving yourself the long-term gift of wellness. You've started this shift by developing new thoughts and beliefs, an internal perspective of your health and wellness, and a new identity—your *Wellness Vision*. Your *Lifestyle Wellness Strategic Plan* brings your *Wellness Vision* to life; it demonstrates you are serious about investing in your wellness and defines how you optimize the return on your investment by living a balanced, health-promoting, disease-free lifestyle. Similar to a strategic plan you would use for a business endeavor, your *Lifestyle Wellness Strategic Plan* shapes the specific tactics and investments you'll undertake to achieve the mission and vision you've developed for your wellness journey. The first four sections of your plan are analogous to a travel brochure for your lifestyle wellness journey. Imagine your *Wellness Vision* on the cover of a tri-fold brochure. Inside, you see images that depict why you want to embark on your journey, highlighted prominently by the name of your road to change. Your supporting strengths and list of pros for change read like incredible comforts, features, and benefits you get to experience. Next, you see images and more information about the goals, attractions, and activities to enhance your journey. You get the picture; it sounds like a fantastic journey. I look forward to seeing you there!

In the remaining chapters, guided by these four sections, you get to create tactics and distractions to initiate your lifestyle wellness journey and strategies to continue and sustain your Well-Leader Mindset™ strategic progression. You will face challenges along the way to giving yourself the gift of wellness. However, you will have already thought through potential challenges you may face, identified their triggers, and determined how you get to manage your thoughts around these challenges. Your tactics and strategies focus on *what you decide to do with what you are given*. It's not about finding the silver lining, thinking positively, suppressing your feelings, or calling on willpower. It's about accepting and managing your own thoughts and feelings when challenges occur, working through them, and acting on what you believe and can control: your thoughts, beliefs, and actions. I'm sending you energy and excitement about getting started on the adventure you've outlined in your wellness travel brochure. You will soon be ready to turn the corner and experience *authentic wellness*. Ready, Set, almost a Go!

Strategic Wellness Activities

You will document the first four sections of your *Lifestyle Wellness Strategic Plan* using inputs from the previous chapters' activities. Compiling the first four sections of your *Lifestyle Wellness Strategic Plan* gives you time to review, reflect, and reorganize your foundational work. Also, it provides an opportunity for you to make adjustments before you get to the detailed planning. Take the time to review and update your foundational work; this guides your next steps and actions.

1. **Download the *Lifestyle Wellness Strategic Plan* template.**

   You will use this template to enter the key inputs you've developed thus far as well as enter your planning work for the remaining chapters. The plan template is located on the book resource website. Follow the instructions and process in the guide to compile your plan.

2. **Complete Section 1.0: My Wellness Mission, Vision, and Aspirations.**

   This section presents your overall presentation of why you want to embark on your wellness journey (*Wellness Why*), your aspirations (road-to-change name), and what you envision you get to become (*Wellness Vision*).

3. **Complete Section 2.0: My *Wellness Authenticity.***

   This section highlights the core strengths and values that will guide your day-to-day and long-range decision-making about your health choices. Enter your top five strengths and how you will leverage them to support your strategic wellness journey.

4. **Complete Section 3.0: My *Wellness Presence.***

   This is your RICE Analysis. These four components support your ability to stay focused and motivated along your strategic health and wellness journey. Enter your current RICE ratings, determine how you will detect an imbalance, and then identify tactics to keep all components in balance.

5. **Complete Section 4.0: My Lifestyle Wellness Investment Goals & Targets.**

   This section organizes and presents your *Current Baseline* and *Future Target* ratings for all lifestyle wellness components and your *Overall Lifestyle Wellness* ratings. You concentrate on and align your tactics and distractions with your targets to bring your *Wellness Vision* to life. You may decide to add *Interim Goals* for components with larger gaps. Bridge goals feel more realistic and keep your plan feeling doable and authentic. When in doubt, choose slow and steady.

6. **Complete the Courage & Confidence Check.**

   Your belief in the completeness of the foundational components of your plan impacts your courage and confidence to move forward. It's not always easy to pause to view your health and wellness from a strategic, long-term, internal perspective. When you review your goals and targets, you must accept that your current actions may be inciting and accelerating chronic diseases of lifestyle and unhealthy aging in your body. You have committed to changing that. Your plan supports your new beliefs and builds a strong case for realizing your *authentic wellness*.

The choices you make daily that impact your health and wellness in the long term are guided by the foundational components of your plan. Your *Future Targets* reflect your investment decisions about how you want to live into the future—potentially disease-free (green range) or taking chances with your genetics and managing chronic diseases of lifestyle with medications, doctor's visits, and procedures (red-yellow range). Your *Willingness to Invest* enough to potentially move and sustain your wellness practices into the green range may increase the probability your tactics add years to your life and life to your years.

The key here is to think about your long-term *Future Targets* as what you *authentically* believe for your health and wellness and what you feel confident you can, and you will continue to achieve, maintain, and sustain into the future. In Part 3, you begin planning your tactics and distractions based on what it looks like to achieve the *Future Targets* you've set. You may decide to start a 6-month *Interim Goal* to bridge larger gaps between your *Current Baseline* and *Future Target* for some lifestyle wellness components. You then adjust and balance your actions to align with your *Interim Goal* as you work toward achieving your *Future Target*. No worries—you can always modify your goals and targets again later if necessary. This is your plan. It must fit your life!

WLM in Practice

Haley wanted to do enough to potentially reverse her chronic diseases of lifestyle. She rated her *Current Baseline* for the movement component at 10 percent and, being the high achiever she is, set her *Future Target* at 100 percent. She contracted with her neighbor, a personal trainer who engaged her in intense, high-impact training three days per week. Unfortunately, the trainer progressed Haley too quickly, which aggravated her knee injuries. As a result, Haley canceled her training sessions and was back to square one. After her knee injuries had resolved and her medical provider cleared her, we worked together to shift her high-achiever mindset to believe in and accept a slower progression toward her *Future Target* of 100 percent. She continued progressing, staying consistent with her *Interim Goal* for movement of 40 percent using low-impact activities spread throughout her busy day.

Sheila wanted to do enough to potentially reverse her heart disease and high blood pressure. She rated her *Current Baseline* for the Nutrition component at 20 percent. Initially, her *Future Target* auto-calculated to be 90 percent, which moved her into the green range. At this level, her actions may have the potential to prevent and reverse her chronic diseases of lifestyle. This was a significant gap to close; however, she was highly committed to investing in her long-term *Future Target* and motivated to work with her medical provider to reduce her medication requirements. Sheila worked on shifting her mindset to think and believe forward. She believed patience and consistency would get her there. She decided to set her first 6-month *Interim Goal* for Nutrition at 50 percent.

✦ ✦ ✦

Stick with me. This will all come together for you soon. Essentially, you are balancing the evidence-based lifestyle medicine practices you get to implement to achieve your long-term *Future Targets* by using shorter-term *Interim Goals*. This balancing process gives you control. You get to make informed decisions about how to live your *Wellness Vision* in a way that feels authentic in your current lifestyle as you progress toward your *Future Targets*. Because Sheila had active chronic diseases of lifestyle and was on medications, she required close monitoring by her medical provider. To experience the outcomes she desired, she would most likely have to do more over a longer duration because research supports that the prevention of chronic diseases of lifestyle may require fewer changes than would be necessary to potentially achieve reversal.

Clients have told me that the balancing and aligning process is the most eye-opening component of their *Lifestyle Wellness Strategic Plan* development experience; it's a completely different perspective than what they've used in the past. Traditional health and wellness tend to take an external approach, focusing on how we look on the outside versus how we are caring for or beating up our internal organs. In the next chapters, you begin transitioning into the detailed planning process; you now get to see what each level (red-orange-yellow-green) of my theoretical chronic disease progression continuum looks like for your *Future Targets*. The detailed planning process provides another opportunity for you to adjust your *Future Targets*. You get to decide to do more or start with less. I created the levels and associated percentages of healthy behaviors using evidence-based standards and guidelines recommended by the American College of Lifestyle Medicine and supporting health organizations. Just as you did with your *Wellness Vision*, picturing what the tactics look like at each level helps you decide how much change feels authentic now and if you are motivated to invest more to begin your transition. Your success is linked to starting with what works for you now. Don't bite off more than you can chew, and don't start with too little. You can adjust and build on that in the future.

The remaining six sections in your *Lifestyle Wellness Strategic Plan* focus on the active components of your plan—the tactics and distractions you get to invest in as you work toward your *Future Targets*. Action is typically where health and wellness programs and solutions begin. However, the *Lifestyle Wellness Strategic Plan* development process is unique. The focus is on mindset change first and then the long game, or, in other words, the "life game," not what you can achieve in thirty, sixty, or ninety days, or even six months. Instead, it's about taking control of your health and wellness destiny now and sustaining it long into the future by transforming your mindset into that of a strategic wellness investor and adopting an internal perspective of health and longevity.

When you complete your plan, you will be able to envision how your decisions and choices potentially affect the functioning of your body systems and how they may influence chronic disease progression (red-yellow-green). You get to make informed choices to balance the life or death-by-chronic-lifestyle-disease decisions that align with your *Future Targets*, so you experience your *Wellness Vision*—no more *shoulding* and *shouldn'ting*, no more wellness cognitive dissonance. And, possibly as I did, after a period of making healthy choices and feeling great, I could tell the difference in how my body responded when I chose the less-than-healthy options, further motivating me to continue investing in my wellness. How will you choose to live out your life? By taking the stay-the-same fork in the road with the masses, those who may be knowingly or unknowingly inciting and accelerating chronic diseases of lifestyle, or by taking the road-to-change fork less traveled. You get to choose to be the well-leader and *healthy disruptor* like I did—the strategic wellness investor who takes control by potentially preventing and reversing chronic diseases using lifestyle medicine. Full transparency: the road less traveled is not always easy and popular, nor is standing out as the disruptor. However, when you have the courage and confidence to achieve *authenticity*, I guarantee there's no better feeling.

When your plan is complete, you will have the tools to become the disrupter and add years to your life and life to your years. The choice is yours every day! Your *Lifestyle Wellness Strategic Plan* will be ready to implement when you are prepared to begin your strategic wellness journey. You get to be creative now and leverage your strengths and values to develop the tactics and distractions to achieve your goals and targets. Then you determine how to measure your progress toward optimizing your wellness investment, build resilience to sustain your momentum, and enhance and stabilize your readiness, importance, confidence, and enthusiasm throughout your lifetime wellness journey.

Dr. Lori's Insights

- It's time for your new beginning—time for a release of energy in a new direction toward achieving your best self. The choice is yours every day!
- Your focus is now the *long game*, and about you taking control of your health and wellness destiny—taking an internal perspective and one of health and longevity. It's about looking at how what you do now may impact the health of your body systems and about you making informed, life or death-by-chronic-disease decisions every day!
- Becoming a strategic wellness investor quiets the mindset struggle and tug-of-war in your brain. You get to live your best life your way effortlessly.

CHAPTER THIRTEEN

The Lifestyle of Wellness Investing

Lifestyle wellness investing enables you to take control of your health and wellness destiny in the present by shifting your focus to the long-life game. You get to stop living the same year over and over, waiting for chronic diseases of lifestyle to set in. Instead, you optimize your wellness investments, which may compound daily to potentially add years to your life and life to your years. When you become a strategic wellness investor, you are no longer at the mercy of your genetics. As a leader, you invest in your business daily, weigh the available evidence, consider internal and external perspectives, and then make decisions. Your *Lifestyle Wellness Strategic Plan* integrates best practices and available evidence so you get to make informed decisions about your health and wellness destiny based on what fits your lifestyle. There is no need for perfection; I rarely achieve 100 percent on all components. However, staying updated on evidence-based practices helps me choose accordingly, being fully aware of the implications of my choices.

I find it interesting that people invest in their careers to achieve success and in their wealth over the years to ensure they have enough for retirement and leave a legacy, yet they are often willing to invest in their health only after it has been devastated. I'm thankful I experienced my wake-up call before this happened, and I am hopeful the same is true for you. As a result, I decided to stop squandering the health and longevity that runs in my family and avoid using my wealth to pay for medications, procedures, therapy, higher health insurance premiums, support, and equipment. Developing your Lifestyle Wellness Strategic Plan supports treating your health like wealth by accepting that it may take extra time and effort today, but know that it is worth it because of the return on that investment tomorrow. However, by getting healthy now, there is no need to wait until tomorrow to pass on your health and wellness legacy. You pass on your legacy now!

You've done great work thus far completing the first four sections of your plan, which serve as your beacon for where you get to go and what you envision for your best self. These sections—especially Section 4.0—will guide the wellness investments you choose to get you there. This is the point in your planning where you shift from the *what* to the *how*. I am pretty sure it's what you've been waiting for. Unfortunately, most programs begin by going straight to the how and that's why they may fail for most people. Going straight to the how without first taking time for mindset transition leads to failure in the long term or simply doing more of the same that didn't work the first time. However, when you understand what motivates you to give yourself the gift of wellness now, what that looks like, and what will make the journey feel authentic, you can't help but be successful in choosing the *how* this time.

The next section of your plan: Section 5.0: My Lifestyle Wellness Investor Mindset Tactics & Distractions helps you begin to prioritize the areas in which you invest when you are ready to implement your plan. You may choose to set 6-month *Interim Goals* or bridge goals to start. Significant gaps tend to reduce motivation because your brain recognizes that the gap may seem unrealistic or insurmountable. I suggest setting an *Interim Goal* when the gap between your *Current Baseline* and *Future Target* is greater than 20–25 percent. It's entirely up to you, however. Setting bridge goals help reduce dissonance; they allow you to practice making progress toward your *Future Target* and validate in your mind that your journey is believable and doable.

You will use the following steps in the next three chapter's strategic wellness activities to select your wellness investments for each component:

1. Review the *Evidence-Based Quality Standard* (*EBQS*) for each lifestyle wellness component.
2. Use your *Interim Goal*, if you've set one or your *Future Target*, to determine the percentage of evidence-based lifestyle medicine tactics required to meet the components of the standard.
3. Choose your tactics and distractions aligned with your strengths and values that will work for you to achieve your goal or target percentage.
4. Experiment and adjust as necessary. Don't hesitate to review and adjust your *Interim Goals* until you believe things feel doable for you in the present. This is an essential step.

Your *Interim Goals*, *Future Targets*, and *EBQSs* for each lifestyle wellness component integrate to provide clear, specific, positive intentions you get to use to optimize your wellness investments. These intentions support your belief that you can, and you will create the new you—the you who treats health as an important wealth.

I provided a brief description of lifestyle medicine in an earlier chapter. However, before you move forward with choosing your wellness investments, I think it would be a great time to take a deeper dive into the basics of lifestyle medicine. Lifestyle Medicine as promoted by the American College of Lifestyle Medicine (ACLM) may be a new concept to you. You already know your lifestyle choices and habits impact your health and wellness, but you may not know that there is a formal, physician-led organization that provides standards, education, resources, community, and board certification in lifestyle medicine for physicians and other health professionals. ACLM is the nation's medical professional association for physicians, allied health professionals, healthcare executives, and those in professions devoted to transforming health and redefining healthcare through lifestyle medicine.[20] Lifestyle medicine uses evidence-based approaches to address chronic disease by replacing unhealthy behaviors with positive behaviors in six areas:

- Healthful Eating
- Increased Movement
- Improved Sleep
- Managing Stress
- Avoiding Risky Substances
- Developing Positivity & Maintaining Social Connections

Lifestyle medicine practitioners encourage patients and clients to become more engaged, active participants in their self-care to impact their disease prevention and management and improve their overall well-being, often without pills and procedures. Your *Lifestyle Wellness Strategic Plan* provides the framework for you to become an intentional and active participant in your health and wellness versus staying reactive, simply going along with mainstream, reductionist thinking and hoping for the best. Throughout the remainder of the plan development process, and as you further refine your goals, targets, tactics, and distractions for each lifestyle wellness area, you learn more about these six components, plus how to create home and work environments that support the implementation of your plan. Without supportive and safe environments, it is an uphill battle to implement lifestyle medicine and achieve the health and wellness you desire.

As you complete Section 5.0 of your plan, you get to see what your tactics look like to align with your *Interim Goals* and *Future Targets*. For example, what does a Movement *Future Target* of 60 percent look like? You will visualize it. The percentage and color level on my chronic disease

---

[20] American College of Lifestyle Medicine, *"What is Lifestyle Medicine?"*

progression potential continuum and how your tactics at that level may affect your chronic disease development ensures you make informed decisions about what it will take to achieve your desired health and wellness. How does it feel to know you will have the ability to actively adapt and adjust your efforts to potentially control your health and wellness destiny? This is the true power of having a *Lifestyle Wellness Strategic Plan.*

I suggest you take a moment to review the completeness of the first four foundational sections of your *Lifestyle Wellness Strategic Plan.* Next, examine the gaps between your *Current Baseline* and *Future Target* ratings; this will help you prioritize the components you choose to work on first. You may want to think about creating 6-month *Interim Goals* for components with larger gaps—you get to decide the speed of your progression. Your decisions will guide your wellness investments—the tactics and distractions that work for you, your custom *how to.* Because of the integrated nature of all the lifestyle wellness components, the most effective wellness investment strategy concurrently addresses all six lifestyle medicine components to some degree. Also, changing your home and work environments often accelerates optimization of your investment return and impact toward achieving your *Overall Lifestyle Wellness Future Targets.*

You've learned that therapeutic lifestyle interventions benefit almost all conditions, as well as symptoms not generally considered a condition. However, *underdosing* of lifestyle interventions is a common problem in healthcare today and may contribute to providers and patients feeling as though lifestyle changes don't work. *You must make enough change to move the needle or scale back your expectations to match your effort level.* This is an important concept to keep at the forefront; it is often the reason people get bored or give up on their health and wellness goals and is a great source of wellness cognitive dissonance. Some of your lifestyle wellness components may have smaller gaps between your *Current Baseline* and *Future Target* or no gap at all. You may feel compelled to make more significant changes for the other components and work toward closing larger gaps using 6-month *Interim Goals.*

You can choose to continue down the same path and potentially face chronic diseases of lifestyle treated with doctor's visits, procedures, and pills with potential side effects. Or you can choose to take an active role in potentially arresting, reversing, and preventing chronic diseases of lifestyle by becoming a *savvy wellness investor.* Which path do you think most people select, knowingly or unknowingly? For me, believing and living in a way that gives me the power to potentially prevent and reverse chronic diseases of lifestyle elicits a feeling of extreme excitement. I am a bit of a self-control freak, as are many leaders! I hope you feel the same. So take a moment to consider the gravity of the next series of decisions you are getting ready to make—the *life-changing wellness investment decisions* that get to make up your *how.*

Strategic Wellness Activities

In previous chapters' strategic wellness activities, you identified your *Current Baseline, Desired Goal,* and *Willingness to Invest* for each lifestyle wellness component. Your *Desired Goals* and *Willingness to Invest* ratings created your initial composite *Future Targets* to make your *Wellness Vision* a reality. Your long-range *Future Targets* typically have time horizons of at least a year (most likely longer); however, starting with what you *believe* you can consistently and realistically achieve within a sixmonth planning horizon is best. Based on your ratings and targets, if you have a gap of 20–25 percent or less between your *Current Baseline* and your *Future Target* and believe you can realistically work toward and sustain it in six months, then your 6-month *Interim Goal* for that component will be your *Future Target*. No need to set an *Interim Goal* unless you still believe smaller increments will feel more authentic for you. Before you move on to the detailed planning, review your goals and targets to ensure you believe your plan feels authentic and doable within the context of your current lifestyle. In Part 3, you continue to drill down to create specific tactics and distractions to achieve your goals and targets.

1. **Set 6-month *Interim Goals* for each lifestyle wellness component.**
   Return to Section 4.0 in your *Lifestyle Wellness Strategic Plan*. For each lifestyle wellness component, read the *EBQS*, examine the gap between your *Current Baseline* and *Future Target*, and set a 6-month *Interim Goal*. Follow the instructions and process in the guide to set your goals. You may decide to readjust your goals and targets again when you begin detailed planning in Part 3. Nothing is set in stone; iteration and experimentation are the keys to achieving authenticity.

2. **Complete the Courage & Confidence Check.**
   Your courage and confidence affect where you set your 6-month *Interim Goals* for each lifestyle wellness component based on your awareness of the *EBQSs* and the level of change you decide to make. You will learn more about the attributes of each standard in the following three chapters and what feels authentic for you; however, it's not always easy to predict the future—life has a way of interrupting even the best-laid plans.

You are simply choosing a starting point. When developing your *Interim Goals*, don't take on more than you can handle right now. Sometimes a smaller, realistic, and achievable goal will help you get started on a more positive note. Also, achieving and sustaining some of your longrange *Future Targets* may take time and additional six-month goal iterations for you to transition effectively and achieve your targets fully. That's why you should think of your *Lifestyle Wellness Strategic Plan* as a living, breathing document that you review periodically and update as you achieve interim targets and when your life situation changes. It may work best for you to focus on some of the components fully and make smaller changes in other areas. All lifestyle wellness components are interrelated. For example, research supports that improving your sleep, nutrition, and physical activity will have an indirect, positive effect on your mood and stress management.[21]

WLM in Practice

Thinking strategically about your health and wellness from an investment perspective may be new to you. This perspective includes aligning your behaviors with the *Evidence-Based Quality Standard* (*EBQS*) and potential chronic disease progression reduction for each lifestyle wellness component. For Sleep Health, the *EBQS* is more than simply getting seven-to-eight hours of sleep, which many practitioners use as a quality measure. Considering lifestyle medicine best practices, the *EBQS* focuses on improving Sleep Quality by entraining your internal body clock (circadian rhythm) so you fall asleep quicker, stay asleep longer, and awake at a consistent time every morning feeling rested. You get to adjust your investment and design your tactics and distractions for improving sleep quality around these three attributes. The attributes are specific and quantifiable for you to easily align your behaviors with the level that meets your *Interim Goals* and *Future Targets*. In the following chapters, you get to align your tactics and distractions for each lifestyle wellness component. It's up to you to tailor your tactics to support your *Wellness Vision* and align with your core strengths, so your plan always feels authentic to you. I provide some guidance to get you started; however, don't think about what other people are doing, what you think you should be doing, or compare yourself to some arbitrary standard. It's about you this time.

Aligning your goals and targets with your expectations about what can be achieved using evidence-based lifestyle medicine practices is the way to eliminate the wellness cognitive dissonance you may be experiencing. It's what I used then and still use today. By using applied, evidence-based knowledge, you get to have the power to influence, redefine, and redirect your wellness trajectory. If your goal is to change your health behaviors to potentially mitigate, stop, and prevent chronic diseases of lifestyle from developing, you must invest *enough* to move your behavioral level toward the green range of the continuum. Currently, my *Future Targets* are all set at 100-percent prevention in the upper green range of the continuum. However, I didn't start there. The table below displays my ratings for Nutrition Health. I rated my *Current Baseline* at 40 percent, and my *Future Target* was 100. Because of the large gap, I chose my first *Interim Goal* of 75 percent. Next, I aligned my behaviors for the *EBQS* quality attributes to work toward achieving at least 75 percent within six-months. After three years, I've consistently achieved 95–100 percent.

---

[21] American College of Lifestyle Medicine, *"What is Lifestyle Medicine."*

Nutrition – Percentage of my nutritional plan based largely on a variety of minimally processed whole plant foods; limited/no meat, deli meat, and dairy products; low added sugar, salt, and oil; low saturated fat, high fiber, and high in fruits, vegetables, beans, legumes, and whole grains.

My Nutrition Current Baseline:	My Nutrition Desired Goal:	My Willingness to Invest to Achieve my Nutrition Desired Goal:	My Nutrition Future Target:
40	100	100	**100**
Rating Description:	Low Healthy Behaviors Low Control/Willingness		Extremely Healthy Behaviors High Control/Willingness

My Wellness Vision (%)			40			75			100

You get to be in control of your investment, how much you choose to control your destiny, and how long you would like to take to potentially influence the development of chronic disease of lifestyle. You may still be thinking, I know my *Current Baseline* and *Future Target* ratings, I see how the level of my current behaviors may have the potential to influence chronic disease progression, and I'm willing to start changing right now. But how do I get started, what do my *Future Targets* look like in practice, and how do I know if I want to invest that much? These are great questions! This demonstrates your thinking is evolving to that of a strategic wellness investor. Stay with me. There is more to come to provide clarity to help you move forward.

You may be feeling a bit nervous or overwhelmed about getting started on your detailed planning. This entire process may seem like overkill. I get it; I've been there. I was stuck in my continuous cycle of wellness failure for over thirty years until I decided to finally change my thinking and treat my health as important as my wealth using wellness strategic planning. Our brains are wired to react emotionally when we are stepping out of our comfort zone or encountering challenges. Both may bring back the thoughts, feelings, and emotions that drive unhealthy choices, procrastination, and negative self-talk. What you practice becomes permanent, so practice overcoming these challenges by acting on the beliefs and possibilities of a healthy you. Stop the cycle! Recognize that these feelings and emotions are normal; I still experience them. Continue using your *Wellness Presence* building activities to overcome the anxiety, limiting thoughts, and doubt that may arise, so you stay future-focused and aligned with your *Wellness Vision*.

It saddens me to think that with all the available lifestyle medicine evidence, 60 percent of adults still have at least one chronic disease related to lifestyle choices, and 40 percent have two or more. People still smoke, overeat saturated fat and processed foods, consume excessive added sugar and salt, don't eat enough fruits and vegetables, and lead sedentary, sleep-deprived lives. Furthermore, 80 percent of premature deaths are attributable to tobacco use, poor diet, and physical inactivity.[22] By moving forward in the wellness strategic planning process, you get to choose to potentially break the cycle in your DNA destiny and reverse and prevent chronic diseases of lifestyle by:

- using evidence-based lifestyle medicine practices to take control of your health and wellness destiny.
- calling upon your *Wellness Presence* often to maintain the courage, confidence, and enthusiasm to prioritize and sustain your plan.
- realizing that lifestyle wellness is a journey of a lifetime—not a destination and then back to life as usual.
- creating your new normal and feeling confident you are making the changes in your lifestyle that are authentic to you and work for your lifestyle for life.

You have reached an incredible point in your wellness strategic planning journey! You've demonstrated that you're committed to investing in your health and wellness and giving yourself this amazing gift. Next, you will enter the creative phase of the detailed planning process. Here you drill down and create focused tactics and distractions to implement the *Interim Goal* you've set for each *Evidence-Based Quality Standard.* This is where you begin to visualize and select your behaviors based on the location of your *Interim Goal* on the red-yellow-green continuum; you translate the behaviors associated with each standard to fit your lifestyle. You will know what 100 percent looks like and what 60 or 75 percent looks like. The key is maintaining your open, investor mindset that you've been cultivating thus far to invent new, creative tactics and distractions that play on your strengths and work for you. Before moving forward, it would be great to take a break and engage in an activity that opens your mind to creativity and endless possibilities.

Dr. Lori's Insights

- If you're not ready to go all in, commit to focusing more on one to two components and less on others to start. However, be sure to make enough lifestyle changes to begin feeling the impacts of your efforts. Don't hesitate to get the support you need to create a plan that works for you. This is your life you are talking about; it's not the time to skimp.

---

[22] American College of Lifestyle Medicine, *"Lifestyle Medicine Core Competencies Program."* mod. LMC1.

- Your body systems are interconnected, and making lifestyle changes in one area affects multiple body systems. Focused lifestyle enhancements can have large effects on your feelings of health and well-being.

- Evidence-based lifestyle changes create a cascade of positive, *healing side effects*; some occur quickly. Therefore, consult with your healthcare provider before making changes to discuss potential impacts on your medical conditions and medication usage.

PART THREE

Your New Life to Live

Welcome to your *new life to live*. You've made it through the messiness of the unknown—the gap between your wake-up call and the beginning of your new way of life. There's no turning back now; you've turned the corner, and the way through to your best self is forward. In Part 1, you prepared the foundation for your strategic wellness journey and reframed your thinking and beliefs about what is possible for your lifelong investment in your *Wellness Vision*. In Part 2, you established your starting point, examined your wellness gaps, and set your initial *Future Targets* and *Interim Goals*. Finally, in Part 3, you get to put the meat (or tofu) around your plan—establish your authentic path forward and how you get to release your new energy and invest in your new life—the one that treats your health as important as your wealth. Your courage, confidence, and readiness to begin your new life will increase as you complete the strategic wellness activities in Part 3.

You've begun your investment mindset shift and have committed to prioritizing your health and wellness, now comes the doing. In the remaining sections of your *Lifestyle Wellness Strategic Plan*, you get to decide what you want to start doing to achieve and sustain the *Interim Goals* and *Future Targets* you've set for your lifestyle wellness components. You will add evidence-based tactics to achieve your goals and targets based on the *Evidence-Based Quality Standards* for all lifestyle wellness components. You choose tactics that leverage your strengths and create positive distractions to keep your enjoyment, enthusiasm, and motivation elevated along the way. Your tactics may include new actions, challenges, processes, and learning events. Positive distractions may include technology devices and apps, group collaboration, support resources, and environment changes. You choose your actions to ensure they align with the standards and that you do enough to achieve your goals and targets. Be ready to experiment; you may feel a little disorganized until you find what works for you at this point in your life. And be prepared to adapt when your situation changes. Life wouldn't have it any other way. Next, you construct basic measurement practices to evaluate how well you are optimizing the return on your wellness investments. I've included a process to track and log your progress to support your continued mindset shift and new perspective of treating your health as wealth—your long-term retirement strategy you get to benefit from now, through retirement, and beyond. Your measurement process helps you stay on track with your wellness goals and targets and provides a means for visually monitoring your progress as you would with your retirement investments. The measurements you decide to include in your *Lifestyle Wellness Strategic Plan* don't have to be elaborate, but they must be enough to provide a high-level overview of your progress to help you adjust your tactics and distractions to sustain your long-term wellness transformation.

You then create your resilience tactics to help you stay focused when your RICE components wane, when you have feelings of self-doubt, and when challenges and life situations arise that could potentially impact your progress on your wellness journey. Thinking about and knowing what could get in the way and how you will proceed before you encounter a bump in the road is critical to investing in your long-term health and wellness. Next, you will determine your sustainment tactics, including external resources and support to keep you moving forward, such as engaging with a strategist or coach, fitness trainer, therapist, nutritional specialist, meal delivery service, equipment, technology, etc. The final two sections of your plan provide an opportunity for you to reflect on your wellness strategic planning process and identify insights and practices you will use to ensure your plan remains a living, breathing document. I've also included a section for you to document insights should you engage with me as your Wellness Investment Strategist to review and support your planning and ongoing implementation of your plan and for sessions and interactions with other expert support resources.

You should expect to feel ambivalent about implementing your completed plan. That is normal, even though you are ready to make changes. This process often triggers old anxieties and concerns about past failures and limitations. That's why your *Lifestyle Wellness Strategic Plan* includes resilience and sustainment tactics to help you identify and manage your feelings and situations that have the potential to affect your commitment. The impact of the actions you've chosen is still unknown and uncertain—are your goals and targets realistic, will you enjoy the tactics and strategies you've chosen, will you have enough support, will you achieve your goals and targets this time? It's unrealistic to think you will have all the answers to these questions now, but after several months of experimenting and doing, you learn more!

You will be ready to implement your new plan when *you feel ready to implement your new plan and not before.* After you complete the wellness strategic planning process, it's okay to step back to take time to reflect, prepare, and gather support before you implement your plan. That's part of the positive transition process; you must believe you are ready and feel ready to act authentically—you believe your plan lays out your authentic path. Also, engage with the resources and support to keep your health and wellness in the forefront and continue moving toward beginning your new life. You've painted an incredible picture of what you visualize for your wellness future, developed your strategic plan, and hired yourself as the CEO of your wellness future. You get to decide what's next. You've done the work; by the end of this planning process, your *Lifestyle Wellness Strategic Plan* will contain a solid plan to invest in your wellness future courageously and confidently!

CHAPTER FOURTEEN

Your Lifestyle Wellness Roadmap—
Eat, Move, Sleep (EMS)

Are you ready to act authentically on your belief that you can, and you will achieve the new healthy version of yourself—you 2.0? Of all the lifestyle medicine components, I feel these three—Eat, Move, and Sleep—are great priorities to start with. That's why I included the acronym EMS in the chapter title, to reflect their urgency and importance. Our bodies crave healthful balanced nutrition, consistent movement, and adequate sleep to perform efficiently, heal, regenerate, and recharge. All six lifestyle medicine components are interrelated, but these three tend to impact all body systems and have the potential to improve your health and wellness quickly (within a few weeks). However, I do not mean to minimize the importance of the other components—avoiding risky substances such as smoking and overuse of alcohol, maintaining positivity and social connections, and managing stress. You work on all these components and supportive home and work environments in the next three chapters. With the exception of avoiding smoking and overuse of alcohol, I believe that starting with significant changes (at least 20–25% increase in *EBQS* behaviors) in the EMS components can significantly influence your wellness trajectory and begin creating a solid wellness foundation for you. Unfortunately, these tend to be the ones people are most resistant to change because habits, culture, beliefs, and limitations have become so automatic and ingrained. However, you now know how to change your beliefs, quiet your limiting thoughts, and mourn the loss of old habits that no longer serve you. You get to structure your life and your home and work environments to give you control over your health and wellness legacy.

I started with the EMS components. I do the cooking for my family and my husband handles the grocery shopping; he also manages the chopping and meal prepping activities based on the meals I have planned for each week. Cooking is much easier when vegetables are chopped and beans and legumes are pre-cooked. We purged our fridge and pantry and changed our food choices to align more with a whole food, plant-based nutritional plan—about 85–90 percent to start. Within two to three weeks, we noticed significant changes—weight loss, normal blood pressure, improved mood, fewer aches and pains, more energy, and improved bowel regularity. My husband's cholesterol dropped 80 points; mine dropped as well but took a bit longer to normalize. We now consistently follow a 95–100 percent whole food, plant-based nutritional plan. It took about three weeks for our cravings to subside and our taste buds to become more sensitive to a variety of new plant-based flavors minus the added salt, oil, and sugar (SOS). After we made the changes, it took two to three years for our whole food, plant-based nutrition plan to heal our bodies internally as reflected by our body composition and biometrics, specifically, reduced inflammatory markers, strong kidney and liver function, and normalized lipid panel (cholesterol, LDL, HDL, and triglycerides).

Experiencing positive health benefits from better sleep quality and more consistent and varied movement took longer to achieve. It took two to three years of being consistent and experimenting with different techniques to increase, achieve, and sustain my sleep quality *Future Target*. I had some kinks and old injuries to work through using yoga, stretching, and low-moderate intensity movement. My sleep and movement components are now in the green range. Was that a sigh I just heard along with, "Really, two-three years?" Yes, but don't feel discouraged—I experienced the effects of the healing long before that. Change your thinking to believe and accept that you have been given this opportunity to achieve greater possibilities! Know that you can, and you will, achieve the health and wellness you desire this time; not tomorrow, not in three months or even six months, but for the rest of your life. You have an amazing life to live.

Along with excellent health, I've gradually *healed* several injuries and have stabilized further degeneration of a neck injury repaired with surgery, using time, patience, and lifestyle medicine. This could be possible for you, too, when you do the work. Remember, it's not a race or a quick fix; you must be willing to step back, make gradual changes if necessary, and be patient. This is what becoming a strategic wellness investor looks like. You get to commit to your lifelong health and wellness journey for the long term. When I say two-to-three years, I mean it took two-to-three years for my strategic wellness investment strategy to shift to autopilot, to become my *authentic normal*. Think about driving a car. You don't have to think about every step; it has become automatic and even enjoyable, just like living your *Wellness Vision* will become. You focus on where you are going and look forward to the journey because the tactics have become second nature.

It's now time to focus on the changes you get to make in all lifestyle wellness components and begin thinking about the tactics and distractions you want to implement. When you selected your *Current Baseline* ratings, were you surprised by how your current behaviors may have the potential to influence the development and progression of chronic disease of lifestyle? What surprised you the most? Unfortunately, unhealthy behaviors become quickly ingrained in your subconscious, occur automatically, and often help you cope or celebrate. You may have become rigidly attached to them. You don't do them because you want to deliberately hurt yourself but may engage in these behaviors to adapt and get you through a certain phase of your life. Fortunately, healthy lifestyle practices and healthy habits are the most important determinants of positive health.[23] You can immediately stop inadvertently hurting yourself. Philosopher Socrates said, "The secret of change is to focus all your energy not on fighting the old, but on building the new." This is the premise of transforming your Well-Leader Mindset™. You get to invest in your wellness using lifestyle medicine practices that not only have the potential to promote health but have been linked to injury and disease-free longevity. Lifestyle medicine is what you use to bring your *Wellness Vision* to life when you take the fork in the road to change. Now let's get started—no looking back!

As I noted in previous chapters, lifestyle medicine uses evidence-based lifestyle therapeutic approaches to treat and often reverse and prevent lifestyle-related chronic diseases that are all too prevalent, such as diabetes, obesity, heart disease, kidney disease, cancer, and the list goes on. According to research summarized by ACLM:

- Numerous studies support that 80 percent of premature deaths are attributable to poor diet, physical inactivity, and tobacco use, and only 3 percent of people in the U.S. practice all four of these health behaviors: not smoking, maintaining a healthy weight, eating five fruits and vegetable servings per day, and maintaining regular physical activity.[24]
- Nearly six million people in the U.S. are living with Alzheimer's disease. Cognitive impairment starts developing at least ten years before a person experiences symptoms of cognitive decline, often due to lifestyle choices.[25]

You may be thinking, *I don't have symptoms of chronic diseases right now.* However, every time you engage in unhealthy behaviors, you may be subjecting your body to conditions that increase your risk for cancer, chronic diseases, and premature death—maybe not today or tomorrow, but repeated

---

[23] American College of Lifestyle Medicine, "*What is Lifestyle Medicine?*"
[24] American College of Lifestyle Medicine. "*Lifestyle Medicine Core Competencies Program.*" mod. LMC9.
[25] Sherzai and Sherzai, *The 30-Day Alzheimer's Solution*, part 1.

exposure may create a higher risk down the road. Your physical health is your *vehicle* for experiencing things that matter most. Invest in keeping your vehicle running efficiently long into your future. The key to health and high-quality longevity is to start where you are now; everything in the past is water under the bridge. So start fresh by using lifestyle medicine practices to potentially stop the progression of chronic diseases and reduce body system disease risk before symptoms appear. You do this by creating a solid foundation in your *Lifestyle Wellness Strategic Plan* and choosing tactics and distractions that demonstrate you are serious about optimizing the return on your health and wellness investments. That's what you will work on in the strategic wellness activities in the following chapters. But, first, it's essential to understand the attributes of the *Evidence-Based Quality Standards (EBQSs)* for Eat, Move, and Sleep, which will help you begin to choose the tactics and distractions that feel authentic to you.

Healthful Eating

The *Evidence-Based Quality Standard* for Nutrition is:

- Optimize healthy, micronutrient-dense food choices using evidence-based dietary practices that include predominantly whole, plant foods that are minimally processed; high in fiber; low in added sugar, salt, and oil; and low in saturated fat.

Chronic Disease Progression Potential	Incite & Accelerate (red)		Slow (orange)		Mitigate & Arrest (yellow)			Prevent & Reverse (green)		
Nutrition *EBQS:*	Less Whole Plant Foods						More Whole Plant Foods			
Rating Range (%)	10	20	30	40	50	60	70	80	90	100

Nutrition tends to be one of the most personal and debated subjects in a person's life; food choices play such an important role, not only for our health and wellness, but socially, emotionally, and even spiritually and culturally.[26] People often become defensive, angry, and *dig in* when their food and drink choices are questioned, or they justify making the choices they do or don't make.

You most likely know maintaining healthy nutrition reduces your risk of heart disease, obesity, diabetes, and other chronic diseases. Did you know research supports that healthy nutrition can *turn off* genetic expression for obesity, diabetes, heart disease, Alzheimer's disease, and certain cancers that may run in your family?[27]

[26] Frates et al., Lifestyle Medicine Handbook, chap. 5.
[27] American College of Lifestyle Medicine. "*Lifestyle Medicine Core Competencies Program.*" mod. N7.

The following thoughts by author Michal Pollan summarize how to use nutrition to potentially slow the progression of, mitigate, and prevent chronic disease: "Eat [real] food. Not too much. Mostly plants. Don't eat anything your great grandmother wouldn't recognize as food."[28] A healthy diet is not overly complicated. The diet part is the overall composition of all your food and drink choices; the healthy part comes down to how often you replace bad choices with good choices. Technically, the better your choices, the healthier you will be, but deciding what is "healthy" is where things get challenging. Applying this using my theoretical model of chronic disease progression, you have the ideal (green), evidence-based nutrition plan, "Eat More Plants," toward the right side of the red-yellow-green continuum, and toward the left side (red), you have the chronic-disease promoting nutritional plan, "Eat Fewer Plants." This means that if you are not eating more plants, you are most likely eating more red meat, poultry, deli and processed meats, dairy products, consuming more sugary drinks, and eating more prepared, ultra-processed foods and snacks containing added sugar, oil, and salt. The closer you get to the ideal, green side of the continuum, the greater the probability your nutritional choices may contribute to preventing and reversing chronic diseases of lifestyle. Basically, you increase the probability of not harming yourself with the food and drinks you are ingesting.

You set your Nutrition *Future Target*. Did you set your target far enough toward the green range to achieve your desired health and wellness? Research has shown that people who adopt overall nutritional plans toward the right side of the spectrum that include predominantly whole plant-based food can experience transformative results in a relatively brief period.[29] The choice is always yours and depends on the results you want to experience. To help you identify your tactics for achieving your Nutrition *Future Target*, it's time to examine in more detail the attributes of the *Evidence-Based Quality Standard* for Nutrition.

Attribute #1: Predominately Whole Plant Foods

What are whole plant foods? You've most likely heard the phrase "plant-based" and now see it on many food labels. An easy way to think about whether a food is a plant food (plant-based) or not is: *plant foods do not have a mother (nor are they derived from the mother)*. Fruits, vegetables, and legumes do not have a mother, compared to meat, poultry, dairy milk, and cheese, which either have a mother or are substances obtained from the female animal. Whole foods are "food as grown," suggesting that when you consume the food, it looks close to how it was when harvested. You can visualize everything that has happened to the food between when it was grown and when you eat it. For example, an apple, a crown of broccoli, and a banana are whole plant foods, whereas apple dumplings, broccoli

[28] DeNoon, "*7 Rules for Eating.*"
[29] Frates et al., *Lifestyle Medicine Handbook*, chap. 5.

powder for a smoothie, and banana bread are not. To determine if an item is a whole food, ask yourself, "Can I pick the item in its current form from a tree, plant, or out of the ground?" If the answer is no, then it is not a whole food. It may still be plant-based or made from plant-based ingredients, but it is not necessarily a whole plant food. Another way to think about whole plant foods is whether you can grow it in your backyard in its current form; I don't think I've ever seen a potato chip bush or a pasta tree in anyone's backyard!

Your body wants to regain its health if you let it. When you don't eat enough whole plant foods, including fruits, vegetables, and intact whole grains, you repeatedly interrupt that healing process. The best approach is to center your diet on whole plant foods—foods that don't usually have an ingredient list. The ideal whole food, plant-based nutrition plan should obtain 90–95 percent of calories from vegetables, fruits, whole grains, beans, legumes, nuts, and seeds, and no more than 5–10 percent from meat, fish, dairy, and eggs. Unfortunately, this is not what most diets look like. According to ACLM, the most over consumed foods are:

- Sugar and high fructose corn syrup found in candy, desserts, yogurt, sauces and dressings, and sweetened beverages and cereals
- Cholesterol found in meat, eggs, poultry, and fish
- Saturated fats found in meats, dairy, eggs, and foods made with added palm oil and coconut oil
- Sodium from commercially prepared and packaged foods such as burgers, sandwiches, frozen mixed dishes, pizza, and soups
- Trans fats typically found in snack foods, candy, margarine, and some dairy desserts
- Processed grains such as white rice, white pasta, crackers, white bread, and foods made with white flour
- High-calorie foods such as butter, oil and margarine and processed meats such as salami, pepperoni, sausage, bacon and deli meats, and snack foods[30]

Consuming too many of these foods contributes to what ACLM considers chronic "diseases of lifestyle." However, research supports that healthful nutrition aligned with a nutritional plan consisting of 95% of calories from whole plant foods and less than 5% from meat, fish, dairy and eggs has the potential to prevent, reverse, and better manage all these conditions:

- Type 2 diabetes
- Cancer

---

[30] Kelly and Shull, *Foundations of Lifestyle Medicine*, 116–118.

- Heart disease
- Kidney disease
- Cataracts
- Chronic Obstructive Pulmonary Disease (COPD)
- Immune function
- Mental health
- Crohn's disease
- Multiple sclerosis[31]

Attribute #2: High Micronutrient Density

Nutrient density is the amount of beneficial nutrients you get from the food you eat. Food supplies both nutrients and calories in the form of carbohydrates, fats, and proteins. Food also contains micronutrients. These do not have calories but are critical for good health. They include vitamins, minerals, fiber, and phytochemicals. The key to optimizing your health and wellness and body composition is to eat predominantly foods that have a relatively high proportion of nutrients to calories; these tend to be whole plant-based items. They are the foods highest in micronutrients and contain antioxidants to decrease inflammation and support increased cell health and immunity, increasing the body's ability to fight infection and prevent the development of disease states.[32]

High micronutrient-dense food families include cruciferous vegetables (broccoli, cauliflower, cabbage), dark green leafy vegetables (kale, spinach, arugula, loose leaf lettuce), carotenoid vegetables (carrots, beets, yams), other vegetables (tomato, celery, squash, peppers, cucumbers, eggplant), dark berries, and other fruits (apples, pears, citrus, melons, tropical fruit). Low micronutrient-dense food families include processed grains (flours), processed sugars, processed fats (oils, dressings, spreads), and animal products (meat, cheese, other dairy products). Think about your current diet; your goal is to stack the deck with high micronutrient-dense foods in place of low micronutrient-dense foods. Expand your diet by eating the rainbow every day—but don't eat the same things every day or every meal. Shoot for twenty varieties of colorful foods every day. Red/orange/yellow foods provide vitamin C, beta-carotene, vitamin A, potassium, zeaxanthin, and flavonoids. Green foods provide iron, calcium, magnesium, zinc, potassium, folate, vitamin K, vitamin C, and vitamin A. Blue/purple foods provide flavonoids, resveratrol, and anthocyanins (dark pigments). White foods provide polyphenols and starches.[33]

---

[31] Centers for Disease Control, "*How You Can Prevent Chronic Diseases.*"
[32] Kelly and Shull, *Foundations of Lifestyle Medicine*, 120.
[33] Kelly and Shull, *Foundations of Lifestyle Medicine*, 121.

Attribute #3: Minimally Processed with No/Low Added Sugar, Oil and Salt & Low Saturated Fat

As described earlier, you should be able to recognize your food and visualize everything that has happened to your food before being consumed. The more recognizable, the less processed the food. You may have heard the terms *processed* and *ultra-processed*, which are not always clear in meaning. There are three levels of processing:[34]

- Level 1: Slightly processed—smashed, diced, or cut with nothing removed (unless inedible). Examples include mashed sweet potatoes, vegetables in soups and stews, and raw cut fresh fruits and vegetables.
- Level 2: Moderately processed—some of the original content was removed and/or mixed with other ingredients available in a typical kitchen. Examples include peeled apples and potatoes, homemade baked goods, smoothies, breads and pasta, rolled oats, and some cereals.
- Level 3: Ultra processed—created in a processing plant, closer to a chemical mix than actual food, with ingredients not found in the typical kitchen such as stabilizers and colorings. Examples of ultra-processed foods are endless in the grocery store and widely available, including but not limited to boxed cereals and meal kits, most prepackaged snack foods, some pre-packaged smoothie mixes, and prepared dessert items. In addition, many protein and energy bars that are touted as healthy also fall into this level of processing.

ACLM recommends that 80 percent of average caloric intake come from whole or Level 1 slightly processed foods and no more than 5% from ultra-processed foods; unfortunately, in the typical diet, 60–65 percent (or more) of caloric intake comes from ultra-processed foods.[35] Processing also creates confusion when it comes to commercially sold foods labeled "plant-based" or "vegan." These are typically meat, cheese, dairy, and egg replacements that are ultra-processed to make them taste and appear similar in consistency by adding salt, sugar, oil, and many unrecognizable ingredients. Consume these replacement foods in limited amounts. When planning your predominantly whole food, plant-based nutritional plan be sure to read the label! Anything beyond Level 1 processing may change the fibrous structure of the plant and offset the health benefits of the whole plant food by adding sugar, salt, and oil. The food may no longer be considered "whole." For example, consider oat groats—the intact grain from the plant—which is considered whole and unprocessed. Level 1 processing turns the oat groats into steel cut oats. Level 2 processing creates rolled oats, quick cooking oats, and oat flour, as long as nothing is removed. Level 3 processing could be gluten-free products containing oat flour. Each level of processing eventually makes the whole plant food unrecognizable and may impact the

---

[34] American College of Lifestyle Medicine. "*Lifestyle Medicine Core Competencies Program.*" mod. NP2.
[35] American College of Lifestyle Medicine. "*Lifestyle Medicine Core Competencies Program.*" mod. NP2.

fiber, nutritional content, and benefits of the food. I am not saying that Level 1 and 2 processed items prepared using whole plant-based items are bad for you. Just be aware that altering the intact nature of the whole plant food has the potential to change the nutritional benefits of the intact plant and your body's digestion and response to the fiber and nutrients in the plant. With processing, the goal is nothing added, nothing taken away, and using ingredients that can be found in a typical kitchen pantry.

Another consideration related to processing is food preparation methods. Certain methods of food preparation increase the formation of advanced glycation end products (AGEs). AGEs are a family of oxidative stress by-products that damage long-living cells in the body (e.g., nerve, kidney, eye, collagen). AGE formation is less when preparing fresh, whole plant foods but can increase significantly in animal-derived foods that are high in fat and protein, such as meats (especially red meats), which are prone to AGE formation through high-heat cooking. Sugary foods and ultra-processed and prepackaged products are also high in AGEs. Cooking methods that increase AGE production are those that use a hot, dry environment such as grilling, broiling, roasting, searing, and frying. Using moist heat at lower temperatures such as stewing, poaching, boiling, and steaming minimizes the formation of AGEs.[36]

Unless you are selecting fruits and vegetables from the produce aisle, reading the nutritional label is the only way to evaluate the level of processing, the addition of salt, sugar, and oil, and the level of saturated fat. Remember, whole plant foods rarely have labels, or the label indicates one ingredient in the package, such as a bag of spinach, lentils, or brown rice. They are minimally processed, high in fiber, low in added salt, sugar, and oil, and low in saturated fat—an optimal food choice. However, if a food item is packaged in any way, always read the nutritional label. Never trust the claims and highlights on the front of the packaging—low sodium, low-fat, organic, vegan, etc. You may have even ignored labels altogether. If you've learned anything throughout this book, you must be more strategic, mindful, and deliberate in your actions. Reading labels helps you make better decisions when shopping and/or cooking for your family and yourself. I love to cook and make just about everything from scratch using whole, plant foods; however, when I do purchase pre-packaged items, I use a few quick, basic steps for reading labels and deciding whether I want my family to ingest pre-packaged food or ultra-processed food-like items. This is not an exhaustive list. It's what my husband and I use so we don't double our time spent in the grocery store reading labels:

- *Minimally processed*—quickly review the ingredients. If the list resembles a short novel, you can't pronounce everything on the list, or the list contains several chemicals, preservatives, and ingredients you don't typically see in a kitchen pantry, it's probably ultra-processed.
- *High fiber*—look for intact grains and 100 percent whole grains, multigrain, and whole

---

[36] American College of Lifestyle Medicine, "*Lifestyle Medicine Core Competencies Program.*" mod. N1.

plant-based items (fruits and vegetables). Adequate intake of fiber ranges between 28–38 grams per day based on a 2,000 calorie per day diet, depending on age and gender. A food containing five grams or more of fiber per serving is considered high in fiber. Choose whole plant foods with natural fiber such as fruits, vegetables, bran, 100 percent whole intact grains, beans, legumes, nuts, and seeds.

- *Low sodium*—it is recommended that sodium intake be limited to less than 2,300 mg per day. A good rule to use to determine if a packaged food is low sodium is to read the label; if the milligrams of sodium per serving is the same or less than the calories per serving, the item is lower in sodium.[37] However, this is true only if you stick to the serving size, and just because it is low in sodium doesn't guarantee the food is nutritious, only lower in sodium. Low sodium potato chips meet this threshold but are moderately to ultra-processed and can be high in fat. Labeling requirements for sodium are: sodium-free is less than five mg per serving, very-low-sodium is 35 mg or less, and low-sodium is typically 140 mg per serving or less.[38]

- *No added sugar*—food manufactures have found endless ways to hide added sugar in foods, such as high fructose corn syrup, molasses, fruit juice concentrate, organic evaporated cane juice, rice syrup, raw sugar, and the list goes on. Fresh fruit contains natural sugars; the concern is about "added sugars." To calculate added sugar, check the label. Divide the grams of added sugar per serving by four (1 gram = ¼ teaspoon). This will give you the number of teaspoons of added sugar (the little packets) per serving. Your goal should be minimal (<10 percent of daily calories) to zero added sugars. Did you know there are almost ten teaspoons of sugar in a typical twelve-ounce sweetened beverage? Artificial sweeteners may not be any better, so limit these as well. Research has shown that continued use of artificial sweeteners may hyper-stimulate our brains to crave more sweet foods and lead to weight gain.[39]

- *Low saturated fat*—this can be achieved by choosing foods higher in unsaturated fat, eliminating or reducing dairy, meat, and other animal products that tend to be highest in saturated fat and cholesterol, and eliminating trans fats (partially hydrogenated oils). For packaged and processed items, avoid foods containing coconut oil, palm oil, soybean oil, and trans fats. Even though these are plant-derived items, research supports that these items negatively impact one's lipid panel.[40] After eliminating foods with these, choose plant-based foods that have less than 20–30 percent of calories from fat. Note that it is easy to confuse percent of calories from fat (which is not printed on the label) with the percent daily value for fat (which is printed on the label). To calculate the percent of calories from fat, multiply the grams of fat per serving

[37] Greger, "*Shaking the Salt Habit.*"
[38] Taub-Dix, *Read It Before You Eat It*, chap 3.
[39] Taub-Dix, *Read It Before You Eat It*, chap 3.
[40] American College of Lifestyle Medicine, "*Lifestyle Medicine Core Competencies Program.*" mod. NP6.

by nine to calculate the total calories from fat per serving. Next, divide this number by the total calories per serving, then multiple by 100. When I used this formula, I found that some of the plant-based food items I was eating had a greater percentage of fat per serving than I thought, so I cut down on the serving size or don't eat the food as often to achieve less than 30 percent of calories from fat overall in my daily nutrition plan. For example, my tofu scramble on almond flour tortillas derives 52 percent of its calories from unsaturated fat. I keep my portion reasonable and balance it with salsa and a bowl of fresh berries. I eat low-fat meals prepared with beans and legumes for the rest of the day. Your goal is to balance your *overall nutritional composition for the week*, not single-meal or food-item specific composition. I've also eliminated the use of cooking oils, and I avoid added oils in pre-packaged foods; however, when I use them or purchase items with added oil, I choose olive, avocado, or other monounsaturated plant oils.

The information in this section and on a typical food label are based on a 2,000 calorie per day diet. It is important to determine your own requirements. The Mayo clinic offers an online tool that considers age, height, weight, and activity level to calculate your daily caloric requirements.[41] You should calculate your daily caloric requirements to determine your macronutrient requirements. Standard recommendations include: protein 10–15 percent of your total daily caloric intake, carbohydrates 70 percent, and fat 15–30 percent. Clients are often concerned about getting enough protein if they reduce or eliminate animal products. You can see from the requirements that most people don't require as much protein as they think.[42] Plant-based protein sources that also contain complex carbohydrates to replace animal sources of protein include all beans (including tofu and tempeh), lentils, other legumes, bulgur, nuts, and seeds; some grains (oats, quinoa, sorghum, buckwheat, cornmeal); and vegetables (broccoli, spinach, asparagus, artichokes, potatoes, sweet potatoes, and brussels sprouts). For complex carbohydrates and fiber, choose whole fruits and vegetables and intact whole grain sources such as brown rice, oat groats, quinoa, other cooked grains, sweet potatoes, and white potatoes (skin on), while limiting processed foods such as bread, pasta, and crackers. Plant-based fat sources include nuts, seeds, tofu, and avocados. Keep your food recognizable and as close to how it looked when harvested. Focus on building balanced meals each week by using plants as the center for main meals, eating all colors of the rainbow, and using whole plant-based items for nutritious snacks; if eating meat and other animal products, demote those to side dish or condiment status.

Important Note *This section provides only a high-level snapshot and is not meant to replace consultation with your healthcare provider and a registered dietitian or nutritionist.* For further resources and tips to start your predominately whole food, plant-based nutrition transition, check the book resource website.

---

41 Mayo Clinic, "*Calorie Calculator.*"
42 Davision, "*The No-B.S. Guide to Vegan Protein.*"

Seek support and assistance from a lifestyle medicine/plant-based aligned dietician or nutritionist for more personalized assistance. Also, after you complete the development of your *Lifestyle Wellness Strategic Plan*, I encourage you to participate in one of my ongoing programs to support the implementation of your plan. My ongoing programs include a full nutritional assessment with planning, maintenance, and tracking using a platform developed and supervised by physicians and registered nutritionists.

Increased Movement

The *Evidence-Based Quality Standard* for Movement is:

- Optimize regular, consistent weekly movement to *achieve total physical fitness* through participating in structured exercise, non-exercise movement, and minimizing daily sitting.

Chronic Disease Progression Potential	Incite & Accelerate (red)			Slow (orange)		Mitigate & Arrest (yellow)		Prevent & Reverse (green)		
Movement EBQS:	Sedentary			Low-Moderate Physical Fitness				Regular Physical Fitness		
Rating Range (%)	10	20	30	40	50	60	70	80	90	100

The human body is designed to move as much as possible. There is no person, including individuals suffering from chronic diseases, whose life would not be enhanced by regular physical activity.[43] You most likely know increasing physical activity facilitates muscular development and growth and increases the synovial fluid in your joints to keep them healthy. Did you know that increasing your physical activity protects and repairs neurons in your brain and increases the production of alpha waves in the brain, which are linked to relaxation and creativity?[44]

Research continues to show that movement truly is medicine. Even Hippocrates is attributed as saying, "… eating alone will not keep [people] well; [they] must also take exercise. For food and exercise, while possessing opposite qualities, yet work together to produce health." It's time to change your mindset to think of physical movement as medicine and as a celebration for what you can do, not a punishment for the unhealthy food you ate. Unfortunately, when working with my clients, some feel that physical activity is a punishment for an unhealthy lifestyle. So, to serve the time for their punishment, they must jump in full speed, join a gym, and exercise at extreme levels and long

---

[43] Frates et al., *Lifestyle Medicine Handbook*, chap. 4.
[44] Frates et al., *Lifestyle Medicine Handbook*, chap. 4.

durations to reap the benefits, or, unfortunately, injure themselves, which usually comes first. I've been there and done that, too! How about you? However, recent research supports that this doesn't have to be the case; a slow, steady increase in exercise intensity is best for health, even if you were active and physically fit years ago.[45]

There is no question that moderate to vigorous physical activity is beneficial to overall cardiovascular health. Again, similar to nutrition, exercise has a dose-response relationship with health—the more physically active you are, the more benefits you reap, *but* any amount of exercise is better than none. There is no threshold level of physical activity that must be achieved before benefits are seen.[46] However, like medicine, it is possible to under-dose and overdose on exercise; more is not always better, so check with your healthcare provider before beginning any exercise program.

What does being physically active mean? Physical activity is any movement of the body done through skeletal muscle contraction that causes energy expenditure beyond your baseline activity level.[47] It is more than planned and structured exercise sessions such as running on a treadmill, brisk walking, or group exercise classes. Instead of focusing on physical activity alone, your evidence-based movement standard focuses on total *physical fitness*. According to ACLM, total physical fitness is the ability to perform one's activities of daily living, respond to emergencies, and enjoy leisure activities with sufficient energy and vitality without excess pain or fatigue.[48] Total physical fitness is the outcome of *general physical activity* (household activities such as stair climbing, cleaning, cutting grass, cooking, standing, etc.) and *exercise* (brisk-walking, rowing, running, cross-fit, yoga, strength training, etc.) to achieve health-related fitness and skills-related fitness, including cardiorespiratory, muscular development, flexibility, body composition, agility, balance and coordination, speed, power, etc.[49] The following table illustrates how total physical fitness (health-related and skill-related) comes together.

Non-Exercise + Structured Exercise = Total Physical Fitness		
Non-Exercise Movement (Lifestyle Activity)	**Structured-Exercise Movement**	**Health-Related Fitness & Skills-Related Fitness**
• Stair climbing • Cleaning • Painting • Gardening • Cooking • Lawn Mowing (walking) • Standing	• Jogging/Running • Resistance Training • Stretching • Yoga • Balance/Agility Training • CrossFit • HIIT	• Cardiorespiratory • Muscular • Flexibility • Body Composition • Agility • Balance & Coordination • Reaction Time

---

[45] American College of Lifestyle Medicine, "*Lifestyle Medicine Core Competencies Program.*" mod. PA2.
[46] Jonas and Phillips, *ACSM's Exercise is Medicine*, chap. 9.
[47] Frates et al., *Lifestyle Medicine Handbook*, chap. 4.
[48] American College of Lifestyle Medicine, "*Lifestyle Medicine Core Competencies Program.*" mod. PA2.
[49] Frates et al., *Lifestyle Medicine Handbook*, chap. 4.

What is the best balance of general physical activity and exercise for you? The best balance for you is the general physical activity and exercise that you actually do regularly and consistently, and it's the balance that works to achieve your desired goals, targets, and outcomes. It's the general physical activity, movement, and exercise you commit to because you enjoy it, it fits easily into your lifestyle, and it doesn't cause injury. The hardest part of regular exercise is the *regular*, not necessarily the exercise. This will be the focus of your lifestyle wellness movement plan—cracking the code to consistency— being creative in order to uncover the physical activity and exercise you can safely commit to doing regularly throughout your day. Start thinking about the activities you already do and what changes and enhancements you can make to increase your activity and improve the regularity in which you do it within the context of your busy life.

You are most likely aware of the benefits of regular physical activity and exercise, including:

- Higher health-related fitness, which means organs and body systems run better, as evidenced by normal biomarkers.
- Easier to control weight and stay at a healthy weight.
- Lower risk of disabling conditions that result from sedentary living, such as bad posture and lack of flexibility.
- Lower chronic disease rates, including heart disease, diabetes, and colon and breast cancers.[50]

But did you know regular physical activity also improves:

- Sleep onset, duration, and quality
- Brain executive function, including concentration, attention, emotional regulation, memory, and your ability to plan and organize
- Symptoms of depression and anxiety
- Perceived quality of life

Immediate results are often seen with a single episode of structured exercise, and within days to weeks of initiating regular exercise, the risk of disease starts decreasing and physical function improves.[51]

For all movement, structured and non-structured, energy expenditure is typically measured in metabolic equivalent units (METs). One MET is the energy exerted (calories burned) per kilogram of body weight for one hour of sitting.[52] For example, a person weighing 150 pounds or approximately

---

[50] American College of Lifestyle Medicine, *"Lifestyle Medicine Core Competencies Program."* mod. PA4.
[51] American College of Lifestyle Medicine, *"Lifestyle Medicine Core Competencies Program."* Mod. PA4.
[52] Compendium of Physical Activities, *"Adult Compendium of Physical Activities."*

68 kg (150 pounds/2.2 kg = 68 kg) burns 68 calories sitting for one hour, versus 5 METs or burning 340 calories for one hour of moderate effort on an elliptical machine. The Healthy Lifestyles Research Center at Arizona State University has compiled an incredible *Compendium of Physical Activities* that provides METs for structured and non-structured activities. I've included a link to their website and a PDF version on the book resource website. You will use this list when you begin planning new activities and think creatively about increasing the MET level of your current activities.

You've set your Movement *Future Target*. Think about your target related to your own total physical fitness. What percentage of your daily movement falls into each category of physical fitness? Did you set your target far enough toward the green range of the continuum to achieve your desired health and wellness? Research has shown that people who adopt balanced movement plans that include all recommended components of total physical fitness can accelerate their transformative outcomes compared to just using nutrition alone.[53] The choice is yours and depends on the results you want to achieve. To help you identify your tactics to achieve your movement goal, let's examine the attributes of the *Evidence-Based Quality Standards* for Movement.

Attribute #1 Structured Exercise

The first component of total physical fitness is structured exercise. Structured exercise is what people typically think of (and dread) when they hear total physical fitness. Many of my clients tell me they get a lot of non-exercise—general movement throughout the day—and consider themselves "fit;" however, without the purposeful, structured movement that causes energy expenditure above your baseline for an extended duration, your total physical fitness may be lacking or out of balance. To achieve benefit, the American College of Sports Medicine (ACSM) and American Heart Association recommend the following health-promoting minimums (for adults under age 65) for structured exercise.[54]

---

[53] American College of Lifestyle Medicine, "*Lifestyle Medicine Core Competencies Program.*" mod. PA4.
[54] Jonas and Phillips, *ACSM's Exercise is Medicine*, intro.

Exercise Type	Minimum Guidelines
Aerobic Exercise	**150 minutes/week of moderate intensity exercise,** or **75 minutes/ week of vigorous intensity exercise,** or a combination of the two
Strength/Resistance Training	**2–3 times per week** on nonconsecutive days; 8–12 reps for each major muscle group
Flexibility/Stretching	**10 minutes; 2–3 days per week;** 2–4 repetitions for each muscle group; holding for 10–30 seconds and accumulating 60 seconds for each stretch
Balance/Neuromotor Training	**20–30 minutes per day**

These are the recommended minimum guidelines to work toward, not what is required right out of the gate. Integrating various daily activities in the 3–6 METs range aligns with the moderate intensity level. Also, the recommendations are cumulative; start with five minutes here, seven minutes there, etc., at work and at home—these short bursts can add up quickly to meet the daily recommendations.

So, you've chosen your activities, so what exactly does low, moderate, and vigorous aerobic activity *feel* like? The *Talk Test* is an easy, subjective measure (see the chart below). If you can still carry on a full conversation or sing, step it up a bit! With moderate intensity, you can still converse but will have to use shorter sentences, take more breaths in between, and will have difficulty singing.[55]

Talk Test: The least objective but easiest measure of intensity assessment.	
Low Intensity	You should be able to talk or sing while exercising.
Moderate Intensity	Talking is comfortable, but singing in more difficult.
Vigorous Intensity	Neither singing nor prolonged talking is possible.

Even though the Talk Test is considered one of the least objective measures, it is quick and accurate enough for most people. When you start, the activity may initially feel more like vigorous intensity; however, after a few weeks of performing the activity, your body systems will adapt, and your intensity rating for the same activity may feel more like moderate intensity. Shoot for a low to moderate range (3–6 METs) to start and work up from there. The same is true for the other components of structured exercise; build up to the recommendations for resistance training, flexibility training, and balance/agility training by finding creative ways to integrate short bursts throughout your day. If this is all new to you, you may want to consider engaging with a certified personal trainer or consult other online support, resources, and books. I've included several resources and links on the book resource website to assist you.

---

[55] Jonas and Phillips, *ACSM's Exercise is Medicine*, chap. 8.

Attribute #2 Non-Structured Movement

Non-structured movement is general physical activity throughout the day, including various non-leisure work activities (e.g., deliveries, lifting, loading, climbing, etc.) and personal leisure and household activities (e.g., stair climbing, cleaning, sweeping, mowing grass, cooking, walking the dog, etc.). To add more non-structured movement into your day, consult the Compendium of Physical Activities list to explore how you can add activities you enjoy with greater than 2 METs, or take your current activities up a notch or two. For example, instead of taking the elevator, take the stairs—stair climbing is 4 METs walking up and 3.5 METs walking down; instead of sitting at your desk for that one-hour virtual meeting, use a standing desk, or, better yet, a treadmill desk like I use. The same 150-pound person described earlier could burn almost two to three times more calories in that one hour compared to sitting. I admit that I was a bit resistant to using a standing desk, and it took some time and practice to get used to it. However, I've since identified the activities I can do well when standing (webinars, presenting, telephone conversations, and online activities) and found that for other activities that require more focus (writing, creative projects, and data analyses) sitting works best. Experiment using standing instead of sitting for different activities at home and work to find what works for you. Give it some time—standing may become your new normal.

Attribute #3 Minimize Daily Sitting

I want to call out this attribute, even though minimizing sitting is somewhat addressed by increasing your structured and non-structured activities. According to the Mayo Clinic, sitting and being sedentary at home and work has become an occupational hazard and serious health risk. Excessive sitting leads to cardiovascular disease, osteoporosis, hypertension, obesity, musculoskeletal pain, diabetes, frailty, weight gain, cancer, and depression.[56] Sitting greater than six hours per day increases the risk of early death by 34 percent in women and 18 percent in men, despite physical activity level; working out once a day at the gym may not reduce the impact of excessive sitting the rest of the day.[57] ACLM presents the following guidelines that outline the risk levels associated with sitting.[58] Think about your average day—what sitting risk category do you fall into?

---

[56] Laskowski, "*What Are the Risks of Sitting Too Much?*"
[57] Laskowski, "*What Are the Risks of Sitting Too Much?*"
[58] American College of Lifestyle Medicine, "*Lifestyle Medicine Core Competencies Program.*" mod. PA2.

Risk Level	Sitting Guidelines
Low	Sitting **less than 4 hours** per day
Medium	Sitting **4–8 hours** per day
High	Sitting **8–11 hours** per day
Very High	Sitting **more than 11 hours** per day

The Mayo Clinic recommends: "Don't sit when you can stand; don't stand when you can move."[59] Still not convinced? This is how consistent excessive daily sitting (greater than eight hours/ day) at work and home wreaks havoc on your body:

- As soon as you sit, electrical activity in the leg muscles shuts off, calorie burning decreases to 1 MET, and enzymes that break down fat decrease.
- After 1–2 days of excessive sitting, good cholesterol decreases and insulin effectiveness and risk of diabetes increase.
- People with sitting jobs have twice the rate of cardiovascular disease as people with standing jobs.
- Women can lose up to 1% of bone mass a year by sitting 6+ hours per day.[60]

Moving more helps your heart and your circulation, increases serotonin to improve mood, helps decrease stress and anxiety, increases energy and productivity, sharpens thinking, boosts metabolism, and builds strong bones, muscles, and ache-free joints. As described earlier, work on connecting movement with the things you are already doing, set a goal to move every hour, and find new ways to move more often and sit less; it's time for a movement makeover!

Important Note *This section provides only a high-level snapshot and is not meant to replace consultation with your healthcare provider and a certified personal trainer.* For further resources and tips to start your movement makeover, check the book resource website. Also, after you complete the development of your *Lifestyle Wellness Strategic Plan*, I encourage you to participate in one of my ongoing programs to support the implementation of your plan. My ongoing programs include a virtual consultation with a certified personal trainer to collaborate on the movement approach and support that will work best for you.

---

[59] Laskowski, *"What Are the Risks of Sitting Too Much?"*
[60] Just Stand.org, *"The Facts: The Human Body is Designed to Move."*

Improved Sleep

The *Evidence-Based Quality Standard* for Sleep is:

- Optimize the quality of your sleep by entraining your internal body clock (circadian rhythm) to reduce wake-sleep time, extend sleep periods, and establish a consistent sleep-wake time.

Chronic Disease Progression Potential	Incite & Accelerate (red)		Slow (orange)		Mitigate & Arrest (yellow)			Prevent & Reverse (green)	
Sleep *EBQS:*	Low Quality		Medium Quality					High Quality	
Rating Range (%)	10	20	30	40	50	60	70	80	90	100

Sleep may be a biological necessity, but optimal sleep is a *learned behavior* that must be *practiced*. Getting a good night's sleep is one of the most important things you can do for your overall health and well-being. Entraining means applying tactics and techniques to modify the phase or period of circadian rhythms aligned to a light cycle.

- You most likely know adequate sleep helps improve brain function, learning, and memory. Did you know getting adequate sleep reduces skin aging, improves your peripheral circulation, and reduces cravings for high calorie foods loaded with sugar, salt, and fat?[61]

One third of life is spent sleeping. Because 60 million US adults have frequent difficulty sleeping, it has become the norm to function on little sleep. On average, most US adults sleep fewer than seven hours per night and feel they can function on less sleep. Research shows that sleep deficiency impairs functional performance, affects mood and motivation, and affects other bodily functions; however, people are often unaware of their level of impairment. There is no recognized objective test for how many hours of sleep a person requires. There are general recommendations of seven-to-eight hours, but there is a considerable range of subjective sleep requirements between people.[62] The standard I created for getting adequate sleep is not to focus on getting a certain number of sleep hours but on getting great *quality* sleep. You feel the impact of great quality sleep in the morning and throughout your day. Great quality sleep looks like this:

---

[61] Frates et al., *Lifestyle Medicine Handbook*, chap. 4.
[62] American College of Lifestyle Medicine, "*Lifestyle Medicine Core Competencies Program.*" mod. SH1.

- When your head hits the pillow, you make a quick transition from wakefulness to sleep onset, usually less than fifteen minutes without assistance from sleep medications or other substances, including alcohol.
- You maintain longer periods of uninterrupted sleep and your body responds appropriately to sleep inputs (I will cover these next).
- You wake naturally after a full night of sleep, within a consistent time range, transition quickly from sleep to wakefulness, and maintain your alertness throughout the day with minimal use of caffeine and other stimulants.

Think about your own sleep patterns. How would you rate your sleep quality? If you rated your quality lower, what barriers are impacting your sleep? Barriers could be related to physical environment, medical conditions or sleep disorders, medications, nutritional factors, alcohol use, life and work demands, and low priority for sleep. It is important to identify the barriers you have so they can be addressed in your *Lifestyle Wellness Strategic Plan*. How can you entrain your circadian rhythm and synchronize your internal sleep processes to improve quality? You do it by adjusting the *external sleep inputs* that affect your quality. The external inputs that affect your sleep quality are:

- daily light exposure intensity and wavelength,
- the food you eat and timing of when you eat,
- the fluids you drink and timing of when you drink, and
- ambient temperature and darkness in your sleep environment.[63]

As you adjust your external sleep inputs, your body responds accordingly. Your sleep quality improves, and you get the sleep your body requires to repair and re-energize. It sounds simple, but is it? Taking control of your sleep inputs can be challenging. When you do take control, adjusting your external inputs affects four critical body responses that promote sleep and wakefulness:

- Core body temperature (temperature of the vital organs of your body)
- Melatonin production by the pineal gland
- Cortisol secretion by the adrenal glands
- Blood flow to the skin (influenced by your hydration status)[64]

These adjustments affect the body responses in the following ways to promote optimal sleep and wakefulness:

---

[63] Kelly and Shull, *Foundations of Lifestyle Medicine*, 261.
[64] Kelly and Shull, *Foundations of Lifestyle Medicine*, 264.

- Core body temperature decreases,
- Peripheral blood vessels dilate to increase skin temperature,
- Melatonin production gradually increases throughout the day and peaks during mid sleep, and
- Cortisol spikes in the morning to stimulate appetite; cortisol then decreases throughout the day.[65]

Therefore, the focus of your lifestyle wellness sleep tactics and distractions is to entrain your internal clock by maximizing the effect of your external inputs. It takes time, patience, and diligence to improve your sleep patterns using evidence-based techniques to change your external inputs. When you commit to making changes, you must stick to the changes for at least three-to-six months, most likely longer, and experiment with what works for you. Don't give up too soon; enhancing sleep quality does not happen overnight, but over many days *and* nights, and there are many moving parts and considerations. Your body will adapt, and your sleep will improve—you will notice when you get the sleep your body requires to repair and re-energize. When adjusting your external inputs, you should address components in these four areas:

- Sleep environment – set sleep routine and times; room temperature, darkness, and noise level; light exposure from clocks, chargers, and nightlights; comfortable bedding, blankets, etc.
- Light exposure – daytime light exposure and activity, nighttime light exposure, screen time and blue light exposure, etc.
- Dietary considerations – timing of meals, daily hydration, caffeine and alcohol consumption, limiting high-sodium foods, timing of high carbohydrate meals, etc.
- Minimizing stress – relaxation and meditation; wind-down routine; warm shower or bath; mitigate worrying, ruminating, and planning; cognitive behavior therapy, etc.

You are in control of these. There are many quick and simple changes you can make that will have a lasting effect. Conducting a quick sleep hygiene self-assessment can highlight areas of concern that affect sleep, such as taking daytime naps longer than 30 minutes; poor daytime hydration; engaging in stimulating activities pre-bedtime; going to bed stressed, angry, or upset; uncomfortable bed and/or bedroom; reading, watching television, or eating in bed; thinking, planning, or worrying in bed; and caffeine or alcohol within three hours of bedtime.

You set your Sleep *Future Target*. Did you set your target far enough toward the green range to achieve your desired health and wellness? Research has shown that people who consistently

---

[65] Kelly and Shull, *Foundations of Lifestyle Medicine*, 265–266.

implement effective sleep plans that focus on all recommended components of sleep quality can improve brain health and accelerate their health outcomes.[66] The choice is yours and depends on the results you want to see. To help you identify your tactics to achieve your health and wellness, let's examine the attributes of the *Evidence-Based Quality Standard* for Sleep and how your external inputs impact each attribute.

Attribute #1 Wake-Sleep Time

Wake-sleep time relates to sleep onset and sleep initiation. Ideal wake-sleep time should be less than fifteen minutes after initiating sleep. Melatonin is important to initiate sleep at onset. Exposure to darkness in the evening triggers melatonin secretion, which causes blood vessel dilation and warming in the extremities and cooling of the body core temperature. Decreasing light exposure at night (blue light from typical household lighting, cellphones, and screens) within one-to-two hours prior to desired sleep time will maximize melatonin secretion and promote sleep initiation.

Also, getting adequate light exposure in the early morning and increasing outdoor activity will suppress melatonin to increase alertness during the day.[67]

Attribute #2 Sleep Periods

Sleep Periods last about ninety minutes and ensure adequate time to cycle through the normal sleep stages (light, deep, and REM sleep) with minimal interruption or fragmentation. Quality sleep occurs when multiple uninterrupted sleep periods occur without waking, or, if you do wake, you fall easily back to sleep. During early sleep, melatonin continues to rise, brain waves slow, and core body temperature continues to decrease while peripheral skin temperature increases. Throughout sleep, cortisol slowly begins to increase in addition to fluctuations in other metabolic components, and DNA remodeling and repair occur. During later sleep, melatonin begins to decline, REM sleep periods occur, and core and body temperature begins to normalize. Similar to wake-sleep time, sleep periods are greatly affected by melatonin production and light exposure. Additionally, bedroom noise and environment, hydration status, meal composition and timing, use of alcohol and caffeine, and stress affect quality sleep periods.[68]

---

[66] American College of Lifestyle Medicine, "*Lifestyle Medicine Core Competencies Program*." mod. SH1.
[67] Kelly and Shull, *Foundations of Lifestyle Medicine*, 267.
[68] Kelly and Shull, *Foundations of Lifestyle Medicine*, 273.

Attribute #3 Sleep-Wake Time

Sleep-Wake time refers to timely, natural transitioning from sleep to wakefulness during a consistent time range and maintaining alertness throughout the day; you don't wake up too early (or too late) in the morning, and you feel rested due to achieving at least six-to-eight hours of high-quality sleep. Upon awakening, cortisol spikes to stimulate appetite, melatonin reaches its lowest point, and core and extremity temperatures return to normal levels. Again, daily light exposure and timing are important, and bedroom environment, increasing evening physical activity, shifting carbohydrate consumption and meal timing, and caffeine intake impact waking and feelings of alertness throughout the day.[69]

Important Note *This section provides only a high-level snapshot and is not meant to replace consultation with your healthcare provider or a sleep specialist.* For further resources and tips to enhance your sleep quality, check the book resource website. Also, after you complete the development of your *Lifestyle Wellness Strategic Plan*, I encourage you to participate in one of my ongoing programs to support the implementation of your plan. My ongoing programs include 1:1 virtual consultation with a certified health and wellness coach to support you and find what works best for you.

Strategic Wellness Activities

The strategic wellness activities in this chapter focus on developing your tactics and distractions in Section 5.0: My Lifestyle Wellness Investor Mindset Tactics & Distractions for Nutrition, Movement, and Sleep. These components nourish your body with plants, enhance your body with movement, and reward your body with rest and regeneration. It's now time for you to determine your tactics to achieve your 6-month *Interim Goals* for these three components and identify any strengths-based distractions to stay engaged and enthusiastic as you move forward.

1. **Complete the *Nutrition, Movement, and Sleep Planning* worksheet.**
   The planning worksheet is included in your investment guide. It explains each *EBQS* in more detail and describes how to interpret and balance your *Interim Goal* percentages and choose the daily, weekly, or monthly tactics and distractions that feel authentic to you.
2. **Reconfirm your 6-month *Interim Goal* percentages and select your tactics and distractions.**

---

[69] Kelly and Shull, *Foundations of Lifestyle Medicine*, 275.

Your tactics and distractions are what you get to use to achieve your *Interim Goals* and *Future Targets* for wholesome Nutrition, consistent Movement, and improved Sleep Quality. Follow the instructions in the guide. See the WLM In Practice section for examples.

3. **Update Section 5.0 in your *Lifestyle Wellness Strategic Plan*.**

   Transcribe your *Future Targets and Interim Goals* for Nutrition, Movement, and Sleep into this section.

4. **Enter your tactics and distractions in your plan.**

   Document the initial tactics and distractions you will use to achieve your *Interim Goals* for wholesome *Nutrition*, consistent *Movement*, and improved quality *Sleep*.

5. **Complete the Courage & Confidence Check.**

   How did you do with creating your tactics and distractions for these components? Do your tactics and distractions for these components reflect your courage to step out of your comfort zone and try new things? How will your distraction(s) keep you on track and motivated? You've learned about evidence-based actions to support nutrition, movement, and sleep— what makes the tactics you've chosen feel *new*, innovative, and aligned with your strengths?

WLM in Practice

Haley set her 6-month *Interim Goal* for Nutrition at 70 percent. She felt that achieving a weekly meal composition consisting of 70 percent whole food plant-based, high micronutrient-dense, high fiber, minimally processed, with low/no added salt, sugar, and saturated fat would work for her. She had two possible weekly options to achieve this: 1) Use the full-meal option by eating three main meals per day (21 per week) and two snacks per day (14 per week) with 70 percent of her main meals (14–15 meals) and snacks (9–10) per week that are whole food plant-based, or; 2) Use the meal-composition option; imagine a pie chart on her plate and add 70 percent whole food, plant-based items, and 30 percent minimally processed meat, fish, or other animal products. Haley decided on a combination of both options; the 70 percent composition option for main meals and shifted to all snacks being whole food, plant-based items. Essentially, she used meat, dairy, and other animal products as a side dish or condiment instead of the main focus of her meals. Some of the tactics and distractions she used to support her 70 percent *Interim Goal* include:

- Selecting an organic, whole food, plant-based meal delivery service three days per week (tactic), so she and her husband could spend more time relaxing together before dinner (distraction).

- Stocking her office with healthy snacks and adding a water cooler (tactic) and keeping the unhealthy snacks hidden to reduce the temptation to grab quick unhealthy snacks when she was busy or stressed (distraction).
- Selecting two whole food, plant-based recipes each week and reviewing them with her husband, who did the cooking (tactic); she subscribed to receive weekly recipes via email (distraction).

For her movement, Haley committed to working toward achieving 60 percent of the *EBQS* for each movement attribute. For structured movement, 60 percent of the recommended 150 minutes per week of moderate intensity would be 90 minutes or, for the recommended 75 minutes of vigorous intensity, 60 percent would be 45 minutes (or a combination of both) per week, 1–2 strength training workouts, 1–2 stretching and flexibility periods, and four days of balance/agility training. For non-structured activities and sitting, the 60 percent of the standard is to enhance non-structured movement to reduce sitting at work and at home to no more than six hours per day. Some of the tactics she used to support her 60 percent *Interim Goal* include:

- walking for twenty minutes (tactic) at lunch with her husband (distraction).
- adding two weekly stretch breaks and hourly standing breaks during work hours to her schedule (tactics); she used her favorite color purple and set hourly reminders on her smartwatch for standing (distraction).
- conducting walking or standing meetings (tactic) to stay energized during long brainstorming and planning meetings (distraction).
- installing an adjustable standing desk (tactic) to stay energized during long meetings (distraction).

For her 6-month *Interim Goal* for sleep quality, she chose to work toward achieving 70 percent of the *EBQS* for each sleep attribute. For wake-sleep time, the ideal time is 15 minutes. Her 70 percent goal would be falling asleep within 30 minutes of sleep initiation. For sleep periods, her 70 percent goal was to shoot for five hours of uninterrupted sleep without extended periods of wakefulness. For sleep-wake time her 70 percent goal was not waking up more than 30–45 minutes before or after her 7:30 a.m. desired wake time (without the use of an alarm). Some of the tactics she used to support her 70 percent *Interim Goal* include:

- eliminating drinking alcohol at night to relax (tactic) and using yoga instead (distraction).
- using a daylight simulating light at her desk to increase daily light exposure (tactic) to offset days when she is unable to get outside (distraction).

- changing the bedroom night lighting to red (tactic) to eliminate blue light exposure at night (no distraction needed)

Nutritional preferences and patterns can be changed. Keep an open mind and experiment with new foods and creative ways to prepare your food. Movement preferences are very individual; what works for one may not work for another. Progress your movement plan slowly and avoid suffering an injury from doing too much too soon—slow and steady this time, and have fun. Sleep behaviors are learned and must be practiced. Sometimes you must *blow up* your evening routine to achieve the sleep quality you desire. Make the easy changes and then use the losing→gaining activity to tackle the more challenging areas. The longer you stay stuck in the past, the more you reinforce and argue for your unhealthy sleep habits. Don't forget to always leverage your strengths to find tactics and distractions that work for you and that you enjoy doing. If you don't buy in and enjoy doing them, they won't stick.

When you live your new beliefs, you push yourself out of your comfort zone, and you *will* feel discomfort. Discomfort is the price of admission to achieve and sustain the health and wellness you desire. Make the decision to choose courage and confidence over discomfort–stop living in the past! Yes, I felt some discomfort. However, for me, the nutrition component was easy; I loved cooking and the creativity involved in taking my old favorite meals and transforming them into healthy, whole food, plant-based versions for my family. We had some major flops, but for the most part they were *keepers*. The more I experimented, the more I willingly invested and stepped out of my comfort zone by incorporating a new vegetable or leafy green into my nutritional plan each month and trying different food combinations.

I didn't expect the discomfort or disappointment I would feel when other family members refused to try my healthier versions or how they seemed insulted when I would bring my own food and not eat the greasy, meaty food they had prepared. Also, what was extremely surprising for me was the sadness I felt when going out to eat and seeing others stuffing themselves full of saturated fat, salt, and sugar. I learned that not everyone is ready to live a lifestyle that cares for and nurtures their bodies from the inside out, even if they are aware. After five years, the discomfort has faded for myself and my family and friends—they are used to me being the outlier and have come to expect my *creative cooking*. They have even become more open to eating and sampling what I've prepared and are enjoying my whole food, plant-based creations. One discomfort has not faded, nor do I think it ever will—the sadness I feel watching people unknowingly or knowingly contributing to the development of chronic diseases of lifestyle.

I treasure my sleep routine and rarely deviate. It has taken two to three years for me to consistently achieve high-quality sleep in the green range of the continuum. I've found my ideal 24-hour circadian rhythm, and I knew it when I found it. Getting to sleep became effortless, and I stayed asleep and woke rejuvenated and motivated. Sleep is enjoyable. I wake up every morning within a 30-minute window without an alarm. I still monitor and evaluate my sleep quality every morning. When I don't feel rested or my quality measures drop, I take time to identify potential impacts from the previous day's activities and things that may have affected my sleep environment (such as forgetting to turn down the thermostat) and make adjustments. Sleep has become a critical component to achieving the health and well-being I desire; I selfishly protect and defend it! It is something I look forward to every night.

On the other hand, I keep my movement plan consistent yet flexible and fluid by integrating my structured and non-structured movement throughout the day. I rarely miss my morning 30-minute mindfulness and creativity session on my WaterRower®. It sets the tone for my day and energizes me on mornings when I rate my sleep quality as a little lower; it also achieves 4.8 METs. Every Sunday, I review my schedule for the week and confirm my movement plan. I get to make necessary changes to fit in my structured activity and decide when I will stand or sit for work meetings. I make other accommodations as needed to achieve my 90 percent target for the week. I focus on standing and moving as much as I can each week and elevating sedentary activities to achieve a higher METs level. Who knew fidgeting while sitting burns almost twice as many calories as sitting still? Feel free to fidget! I don't watch television much; however, after dinner, I walk on my treadmill for at least 30–45 minutes while streaming a video, watching a television episode, or reading. Sometimes I stream videos while cooking and meal prepping, but always moving or standing. How far you want to go with your *Nutrition, Movement,* and *Sleep* tactics and distractions depends on your desired health and wellness *Future Targets.* Do you want to increase the probability your actions are simply slowing the progression of chronic diseases, or would you rather increase the probability your actions are preventing or reversing them altogether? The choice is always

yours—one bite at a time, one step at a time, one snore at a time.

You will complete the remaining lifestyle wellness components in the following two chapters. When you implement your *Lifestyle Wellness Strategic Plan* and focus on your *Interim Goals,* when your tactics and distractions align with your strengths and values, and when you know you are doing *enough* to achieve your *Wellness Vision,* your discomfort fades, and you settle into your authentic new life to live. You place more value on your health and wellness and protect and defend it; you *Eat, Move,* and *Sleep* to *live!* If your discomfort doesn't fade after implementing your tactics and distractions, you haven't yet found what feels authentic to you and what you are willing to invest. You may still be stuck in your old mindset or allowing external expectations from the media and other people to influence your actions and inactions. You may have set your goals and targets too high for where you are and your willingness to invest at that level. That's the beauty of being the CEO of your health and wellness. You weigh the evidence, consider your situation, challenges, and support, then make adjustments and focus on your desired level for the *Evidence-Based Quality Standards* in each lifestyle wellness component. You experiment with tactics and distractions that best fit your lifestyle. Stay courageous; experimentation and practice build confidence. Commit to finding what works for you—making failure *not* an option this time.

Dr. Lori's Insights

- If you're not ready to go all in with your investments, commit to focusing more on the EMS components and less on the other components to start. Be sure to make enough lifestyle changes to begin feeling the impacts of your efforts.
- Strategic wellness investors optimize their health and wellness ROI by aligning their health behaviors with evidence-based standards. This increases the probability that their actions and behaviors are not contributing to the development of chronic diseases—they know how to invest to achieve the health and well-being they envision.
- Craft your tactics and distractions and keep them flexible enough so you can achieve the health and wellness you desire regardless of what is going on in your life and where you are. Always create backup plans to keep you making progress even when you travel or get pulled out of your daily routine.

CHAPTER FIFTEEN

Your Lifestyle Wellness Roadmap– Destress, Connect & Protect

You are well into the action-planning component of your *Lifestyle Wellness Strategic Plan*. Soon you get to implement your plan! I hope you've taken enough time to develop and document concrete *initial* tactics and distractions for *Nutrition*, *Movement*, and *Sleep* in Section 5.0 of your plan. Notice I said *initial* tactics and distractions. Think of your initial tactics as your first experiments. You try them for a few weeks to see how they work for you. I guarantee you will tweak them a bit as you learn more about yourself, your preferences, and what you can integrate into your busy day.

Don't feel discouraged or impatient, this is all part of your lifelong wellness journey. You are in training for life; tweaking your actions becomes normal as you adapt to the new thoughts and feelings you experience as you live your healthy lifestyle. Keep up the great work and never stop experimenting and thinking creatively when developing new tactics and distractions. Avoid the mundane, same-old that isn't working now and didn't work in the past. If it didn't work back then, it most likely won't work now. However, think about why it didn't work; is there a better way to do it? What challenges got in the way? What modified tactics, distractions, and support could make it work this time?

For example, I never liked weight training but loved the results—feeling strong and looking toned. Creating the strength workouts was my husband's department. When he was younger, he trained with a Navy Seal and practiced martial arts. Unfortunately, this led him to create long, extended workouts. I went along at first but always got bored and stopped or made excuses to miss a strength workout. I even reached a point where I hated strength training. Throughout my wellness coaching and lifestyle medicine certification process, I learned about the benefits of strength training for improving cognitive function and enhancing all body systems. I believed I could figure this out and saw my future self feeling strong and looking fit and tone; time to act on my belief. Fact: I got bored with long weight-training workouts, but I like using weights and resistance bands. Solution: I created upper body and lower body routines that take only fifteen-twenty minutes to complete. I use each routine twice a week, usually in the morning, but can easily fit in fifteen-to-twenty minutes later in the day. Short and steady works better for me; I've never gotten injured and have never been stronger—and yes, you can build muscle strength in *old age*.

Nutrition, *Movement*, and *Sleep* create a strong internal foundation for your lifestyle wellness journey. Let's continue to build on this foundation by protecting your body from external influences that have the potential to wreak havoc upon your immune system and increase chronic disease risk for many body systems. The three components I focus on in this chapter are:

- Managing Stress
- Maintaining Positivity & Social Connections
- Avoiding Risky Substances

These may be new areas for you to work on. When thinking about getting "healthy," most people focus only on nutrition and movement and forget about sleep and *everything else* that affects their overall health and wellness. The *everything else* is just as important as nutrition, movement, and sleep. As I mentioned in the previous chapter, your *how* this time *must* be different than what didn't work for you in the past, even different than what did work in the past but didn't stick. So, again, get ready to *blow up* these three areas of your life as you know them, and gather support from family, friends, coworkers, and your community. Working to enhance these areas requires collaboration and support—invest in the resources you need and ask for support this time! Your plan must be different and something you can live with for the long term—kind of like forever. Remember, lifestyle wellness lasts a lifetime.

The information in this chapter may not be new for you. However, did you know:

- Managing stress and avoiding tobacco and alcohol reduce disease risk for all body systems and increase blood flow to the skin and also improves its elasticity?[70]

---

[70] Frates, *Lifestyle Medicine Handbook*, chap. 7.

- Developing and maintaining strong positive connections not only improves your mood and psychological well-being but enhances the functioning of your immune, endocrine, and circulatory systems?[71]

Working on these three components helps you create and maintain a strong internal and psychological foundation for true, long-term lifestyle wellness. I want you to continue to think creatively to come up with innovative and new actions and modify old actions that didn't work. Be sure to align the tactics and distractions you choose with your strengths and values as you did with the first three components. You always have a choice about how you adapt and respond to stress, create positivity and purpose in your life, experience situations, engage in relationships, and what substances and chemicals you expose your body to or choose to put into it.

De-Stress

The *Evidence-Based Quality Standard* for Stress Management is:

- Optimize stress management and resilience using *healthy adaptation and coping mechanisms* to feel in control and experience thoughts and feelings of *increased mental well-being.*

Chronic Disease Progression Potential	Incite & Accelerate (red)		Slow (orange)	Mitigate & Arrest (yellow)		Prevent & Reverse (green)	
Stress Management *EBQS:*	Low Adaptation Adaptation & Well-being		Moderate Adaptation Adaptation & Well-being			High Adaptation & Well-being	
Rating Range (%)	10	20	30	40	50	60	70	80	90	100

Seventy percent of primary care provider visits are related to stress and lifestyle.[72] Experiencing stress is an inevitable part of life; however, it is not the stress that kills us, it is how we react or respond to it. Over forty-three percent of all adults suffer from the adverse effects of stress, and unmanaged stress is associated with poor health and chronic diseases such as diabetes and heart disease.[73] When feeling stressed and overwhelmed, people are less likely to engage in healthy habits, even though

---

[71] Frates, *Lifestyle Medicine Handbook*, chap. 9.
[72] American College of Lifestyle Medicine, "*Lifestyle Medicine Core Competencies Program.*" mod. EW1.
[73] American College of Lifestyle Medicine, "*Lifestyle Medicine Core Competencies Program.*" mod. EW1.

healthy habits can improve mood and reduce stress. Were you surprised by these statistics? Probably not. Stress is a constant in our daily lives at home and at work. No person is immune from stress. Think about what creates stress for you right now. How do you react to it? Do you maintain healthy habits or resort to less than healthy ways to cope with or *numb* the stress?

Stress can be a good thing and a bad thing. The good thing about stress is that it can motivate us to take action to complete a work assignment, a home improvement project, or a workout; it can stimulate our survival instinct (fight or flight) in certain situations as well. This is considered *Eustress*, or good stress. However, when you don't fully resolve your stress, and it remains chronically in the background of your home and work lives, it can impact your health. This is considered *Distress*, or bad stress—the kind that is harmful and draining. What starts out as eustress can transform into distress. Stress occurs at home and work, but what is considered stressful is in the eye of the beholder. Our minds are often powerful instigators of stress. Our thoughts control our feelings, which can impact the body's physiological response to a perceived stress. Stress hormones are released to prepare the body to act in the short term, but if the body is not able to return to a stress-free state, stress becomes chronic with a potential to impact health and wellness.[74]

Just as the perception of factors as stressful varies from person to person, so does the effect of stress on the body. There are non-modifiable factors (genetic) and modifiable factors associated with stress and poor emotional well-being. Lifestyle medicine focuses on addressing the modifiable factors and situations.[75] You may have experienced some, if not all, of these situations that can create ongoing distress:

- External factors such as everyday annoyances, family issues, financial problems, and co-worker and work-related issues
- Internal factors such as excessive caffeine, highly processed foods, insomnia, smoking, and other risky substances
- Physical factors such as illness, injury, pain, obesity, and over-exercising
- Psychological factors such as anxiety, all-or-nothing attitude, perfectionism, unrealistic expectations, taking things personally, and relationship issues[76]

Even though these factors are modifiable, many are unavoidable and possibly out of your control. The important point here is recognizing your feelings and how these factors influence the behaviors you engage in to manage the stress they may cause. When I feel stressed, I experience fatigue, irritability, and loss of focus. In the past, I would try to avoid stressful situations and often reverted to unhealthy behaviors such as drinking wine, stress eating, and binge-streaming videos. I've since

---

[74] Frates, *Lifestyle Medicine Handbook*, chap. 7.
[75] American College of Lifestyle Medicine, "*Lifestyle Medicine Core Competencies Program*." mod. EW1.
[76] Frates, *Lifestyle Medicine Handbook*, chap. 7.

learned to use mindset change practices to step back and examine my thoughts and feelings from a position of neutrality. I let myself feel the emotion. I inform others, if necessary, about what I am feeling, then accept and reframe the stressful situation, choose my new thoughts about the situation, and implement a healthy coping mechanism instead. It takes awareness, practice, and perseverance to stop our normal reactive stress response in its tracks. What effect does stress have on your behavior?

- Do you tend to smoke, drink, or use other risky substances more frequently?
- Do you overeat and make less healthy food choices?
- Do you exercise less frequently, and is the sofa your new best friend?
- What about outbursts of anger, frustration, and sarcasm toward coworkers or family members?

A quick way to assess your perceived stress level over the past month is using a tool called the *Perceived Stress Scale Assessment.*[77] The questionnaire is available on the book resource website. It contains ten items that evaluate symptoms of stress on a scale of 1 (never) to 4 (very often). Take a few minutes right now to complete the assessment. Is your perceived stress level low, moderate, or high? What did you learn about your perceived stress? What areas are causing you the most stress? Understanding the things that increase your perceived stress help you create targeted tactics and distractions to reduce your perceived stress level and move your stress management target into the green range of the continuum. If after completing the assessment you find your perceived stress is high risk, consider contacting your healthcare provider for support.

If stress is inevitable in your life, then what can you do about it? You actively enhance how you control and manage your reaction in stressful situations. Even though some people seem to handle stress better than others, that doesn't mean they don't experience it. They are just better at managing it and using constructive behaviors that help return their bodies to a stress-free level. Don't discount the importance of managing stress for great health and wellness, but it takes time and targeted action to build your stress management capabilities. Stress takes all forms. It is important to identify your stress triggers and develop creative tactics to manage how you think about and respond to stress. Small actions have a cumulative effect. As I mentioned in previous chapters, all lifestyle medicine components are integrated—the changes you make to enhance your nutrition, movement, and sleep directly impact how your body and mind respond to stress and improve your ability to build your stress management capabilities.

You created your Stress Management *Future Target*. Did you set your target far enough toward the green range on the continuum to support achieving your *Wellness Vision*? Research has shown that people who consistently manage stress in constructive ways reduce the probability their actions

---

[77] American College of Lifestyle Medicine, *"Lifestyle Medicine Core Competencies Program."* mod. EW1.

are contributing to their risk of heart disease, diabetes, obesity, and depression.[78] The choice is yours and depends on the results you want to experience. To help you identify your tactics to achieve your health and wellness, let's examine the attributes of the *Evidence-Based Quality Standard* for Stress Management.

Attribute #1 Healthy Adaptation & Coping Mechanisms

Healthy adaptation, coping mechanisms, and self-management relate to implementing techniques to increase the percentage of days that you feel in control of your responsibilities, your reactions to unexpected situations, and your ability to manage personal and work issues that cause stress. Adaptation, coping, and self-management skills include but are not limited to:

- Cognitive-behavioral restructuring
- Mindfulness and meditation
- Breathing techniques and relaxation exercises
- Mindset training
- Assertiveness techniques
- Yoga, Tai Chi, and *flow* experiences
- Spending time in nature or calming environments
- Self-compassion
- Neuro-linguistic reprogramming
- Spiritual and religious activities

Experiment and find the combination of healthy practices that work for you. Many of the techniques in the list are used to cope and manage after your stress response occurs. For example, mindfulness and deep breathing are effective ways to refocus your conscious brain in the present moment. However, these techniques may not be enough to help you reframe the situation to reduce the intensity of your automatic stress response to the problem initially and in the future. I found that structured mindset training was most effective to actively change my thoughts and beliefs about the situation in the moment to minimize or eliminate my stress response. Mindset training is more proactive and effective when you are out there in the trenches living your life.

---

[78] American College of Lifestyle Medicine, "*Lifestyle Medicine Core Competencies Program.*" mod. EW2.

Attribute #2 Balanced Mental Well-being

Well-being relates to enhanced quality of life and what a person believes is intrinsically valuable to them. The dimensions of well-being include the eight lifestyle wellness components and may include career, financial, spiritual, and intellectual satisfaction. In addition, healthy adaptation and coping mechanisms for managing stress and making changes to the EMS components, which are within your control, contribute to greater mental well-being. Examples of these include:

- Nutritional interventions promote positive mood, specifically when you eliminate processed foods and fast food by transitioning to a whole food, plant-based diet rich in fruits and vegetables.[79]
- More movement throughout the day also improves mood by affecting the areas of the brain that regulate our stress response by increasing dopamine in the brain's reward center, which fuels feelings of optimism, joy, and pleasure when connecting with others.[80]
- Better mental health and stress management have been shown in those who sleep between seven and nine hours per night, compared to those who sleep less than seven or more than nine hours per night.[81]
- Courage is another side effect of physical activity on the brain. A new exercise habit enhances the reward system and also increases neural connections among areas of the brain that calm anxiety. Regular physical activity promotes a more balanced nervous system less prone to fight or flight.[82]

Positive mental well-being can be cultivated by:

- acting altruistically rather than being self-centered
- maintaining a growth mindset
- treating stressful challenges as learning opportunities
- building self-confidence
- embracing change
- not sweating the small stuff
- accepting the fact that some things are beyond your control[83]

---

[79] American College of Lifestyle Medicine, "*Lifestyle Medicine Core Competencies Program*." mod. EW2.
[80] American College of Lifestyle Medicine, "*Lifestyle Medicine Core Competencies Program*." mod. PA1.
[81] American College of Lifestyle Medicine, "*Lifestyle Medicine Core Competencies Program*." mod. SH1.
[82] McGonigal, "*Here's How Exercise Reduces Anxiety and Makes You Feel More Connected*."
[83] Kelly and Shull, *Foundations of Lifestyle Medicine*, 242.

You can evaluate your mental well-being using a two-item questionnaire I've included on the book resource website. The questionnaire helps you quickly assess your mental well-being and determine the need for further consultation with your healthcare provider.

Connect

The *Evidence-based Quality Standard* for Developing and Maintaining Positivity & Social Connections is:

- Optimize positivity and connections quality through *increasing your positive possibilities mindset* and *balancing connections* with people, ideas, places, and things that provide meaning.

Chronic Disease Progression Potential	Incite & Accelerate (red)			Slow (orange)		Mitigate & Arrest (yellow)		Prevent & Reverse (green)		
Positivity & Connections *EBQS*:	Low Positivity & Balance			Moderate Positivity & Balance				High Positivity & Balance		
Rating Range (%)	10	20	30	40	50	60	70	80	90	100

There is continually growing evidence that positivity, meaning, and happiness within oneself, developing positive relationships with people, and feeling connected to work, ideas, and places, are essential in mitigating disease risk and promoting longevity.

- You are most likely aware that social connections and positive relationships affect emotional well-being. However, did you know they are the single most important predictors of happiness and longevity and essential to a person's survival and vitality?[84]
- Positive interactions improve physiological function, including heart health and the nervous system's response to stress.[85]
- Positivity and connectedness also benefit the functioning of the immune, endocrine, and cardiovascular systems.[86]

---

[84] Harvard Health Publishing, "*Can Relationships Boost Longevity and Well-being?*"
[85] Hopper, "*How Your Social Life Might Help You Live Longer.*"
[86] Frates, *Lifestyle Medicine Handbook*, chap. 9.

Connections are not only human connections and personal relationships; positive connections can also be with pets, your work mission, beauty and nature, special places, ideas and information, hobbies, a higher purpose, connecting with your inner self, etc.[87] You have a lot of choices in your life about what to do, what to wear, what to eat, and what to spend your money on—the options are endless. However, one choice that people often neglect is their mindset. You have a choice about what to believe and what to think. It's not about sugar-coating and always seeing the silver lining. It's about purposefully choosing a possibilities mindset, changing your perspective, and looking for the positive within ourselves and others. You are setting yourself up for success and happiness. You cannot necessarily choose the situation in which you find yourself, but you can decide what the situation means to you by choosing positive emotions, meanings, and attitudes, including kindness, appreciation, love, joy, open-mindedness, interest, optimism, and relaxation in your life. "With positivity, you see new possibilities, bounce back from setbacks quickly, connect with others on a deeper level, and become the best version of yourself. You even sleep better."[88]

You created your Developing and Maintaining Positivity & Social Connections *Future Target*. Did you set your target far enough toward the green range of the continuum to achieve your *Wellness Vision?* Research has shown that people who consistently engage in and maintain positivity and connectedness achieve greater emotional well-being, health, and longevity.[89] The choice is yours and depends on the results you want to see. To help you identify your tactics to achieve your health and wellness, let's examine the attributes of the *Evidence-Based Standard* for Developing and Maintaining Positivity & Social Connections.

Attribute #1 Balancing Meaningful Connections

A source of positivity in your life can be your connections with others, such as family, friends, coworkers, or group members. To thrive and survive, you need warmhearted connections with other people. Like a vitamin deficiency, a human contact deficiency weakens the body, mind, and spirit. And research even supports that a deficiency in connections may be linked to early death.[90] Don't confuse connection with number of friends, followers, or connections on social media. Meaningful connection is more about feeling part of something larger than yourself, feeling close to another person or group, and feeling welcomed and understood; this could be virtually and in person.

To gain the benefits of connection, it doesn't matter what kind of connections you have. It is the *balance* of connections that is most important. Remember, your connections don't necessarily have

---

[87] Hallowell, *Connect: 12 Vital Ties That Open Your Heart, Lengthen Your Life, and Deepen Your Soul,* intro.
[88] Fredrickson, *Positivity: Discover the Upward Spiral That Will Change Your Life,* chap. 1.
[89] American College of Lifestyle Medicine, "*Lifestyle Medicine Core Competencies Program.*" mod. EW2.
[90] American College of Lifestyle Medicine, "*Lifestyle Medicine Core Competencies Program.*" mod. EW1.

to be limited to family, friends, colleagues, and acquaintances. You can develop meaningful connections at work, home, church, volunteer organizations, or professional or personal interest groups. Even small micro-moments and casual daily interactions with your favorite Barista, restaurant server, cashier, and a brief conversation with the person in the elevator or grocery store contribute to the health benefits of maintaining positive social connections. The key to gaining the health benefits from meaningful connections is balancing your social interactions with maintaining personal space, which can vary from person to person. Some people desire fewer personal connections but thrive on connecting with ideas and places that provide serenity and increase clarity and focus. It's up to you; it's what feels authentic to you.

Attribute #2 Exhibiting a Positive Possibilities Mindset

Positivity and maintaining a possibilities mindset can't prevent all bad things from happening, but may affect the way you perceive the bad things happening to you and how you respond to them. Research supports that positivity feels good, changes how your mind works, transforms your future, puts the brakes on negativity, and you can increase it.[91] However, positive thinking in and of itself will not change your life. You must shift your mindset to support new thoughts, beliefs, and possibilities framed from a positive perspective.

We are human; we aren't supposed to be happy all the time. Contrast gives your life enrichment and depth so you can feel the extremes. Happiness and positivity are about working toward your potential, which demands contrast. You learn more by having to challenge yourself and by experiencing the ups and downs as you work toward your potential. You can achieve what you desire when you manage your mind and process your emotions. Only then will positivity present an opportunity for you to step up to the next level of existence, broaden your mind, and build your best future. From a health and wellness perspective, positive possibilities mindset:

- Protects the heart
- Strengthens the immune system
- Protects against cognitive impairment
- Reduces stress and anxiety
- Improves mood and reduces depression
- Increases longevity[92]

---

[91] Fredrickson, *Positivity: Discover the Upward Spiral That Will Change Your Life,* chap. 1.
[92] American College of Lifestyle Medicine, *"Lifestyle Medicine Core Competencies Program."* mod. EW2.

Positivity is contagious; when you shift your mindset and reframe your thoughts and beliefs using possibilities and positivity, people will notice. Hang out with positive, future-focused people or be the source of positivity in your life and interactions.[93] Developing & Maintaining Positivity & Social Connections are important therapeutic lifestyle changes that promote physical health and mental and emotional well-being. Decide to move your life forward in a positive direction, believe and act on your possibilities and purpose, and make time to create meaningful connections with others; it's good for your health.

Protect

The *Evidence-based Quality Standard* for Risky Substance Avoidance is:

- Optimize a substance management strategy by *avoiding alcohol use* and *elimination of tobacco and other risky substances.*

Chronic Disease Progression Potential	Incite & Accelerate (red)		Slow (orange)		Mitigate & Arrest (yellow)			Prevent & Reverse (green)	
*Risky Substance Avoidance *EBQS:*	High Risk/ Bing		Low Risk			Rare Use			Full Avoidance
Rating Range (%)	10	20	30	40	50	60	70	80	90	100

*Note: Model for Alcohol use only. Full elimination of smoking and other substance use is recommended.

The use of risky substances such as alcohol, tobacco, and recreational drugs, increases your risk of many chronic diseases and death.

- You are most likely aware that the use and overuse of alcohol and tobacco products are the top causes of chronic diseases and preventable deaths in the United States. Did you know that use of these substances weakens your immune system and your ability to fight off infection?[94]

People are prone to overusing a wide variety of substances, ranging from food to drugs, with the most common being alcohol, tobacco, cannabis, stimulants, and opioids. Overuse of any of these

---

[93] Fredrickson, *Positivity: Discover the Upward Spiral That Will Change Your Life,* chap. 4.
[94] Frates, *Lifestyle Medicine Handbook*, chap. 11.

substances is now referred to as substance use disorder, which occurs when the person's recurrent use of alcohol and/or drugs causes clinically and functionally significant impairment at work, school, or home.[95] Think about your own patterns of use for these substances, why you use them, and if you feel there may be times when you tend to overuse any of them.

You created your Risky Substance Avoidance *Future Target*. Did you set your target far enough toward the green range of the continuum to support your *Wellness Vision*? To help you identify your tactics to achieve your health and wellness, let's examine the attributes of the *Evidence-Based Quality Standard* for Risky Substance Avoidance.

Attribute #1 Avoiding Alcohol Use

Statistics indicate that alcohol is the most widely used substance in the United States. In fact, 86 percent of people ages eighteen or older have ingested some type of alcohol, with at least 70 percent consuming alcohol within the past year.[96] Effects of alcohol on health and longevity include:

- High blood pressure and stroke
- Fatty liver, cirrhosis, and hepatitis
- Pancreatitis
- Weakened immune system
- Increased risk of developing certain cancers[97]

The National Institutes of Health (NIH) provides the following guidelines for alcohol use.[98] The drink limits are lower for women due to lower body weight and blood volumes less than males. Thirty percent of US adults exceed the daily limits presented in the following table. NOTE: Achieving the NIH guidelines places you at 30 percent on my red-yellow-green continuum for this component because there is mixed evidence on the use of alcohol pointing to the health benefits of reducing it as much as possible, showing that even light to moderate drinking has been associated with shrinking in the areas of the brain associated with cognition and learning.[99]

---

[95] American College of Lifestyle Medicine, "*Lifestyle Medicine Core Competencies Program.*" mod. AU1.
[96] American College of Lifestyle Medicine, "*Lifestyle Medicine Core Competencies Program.*" mod. AU1.
[97] Kelly and Shull, *Foundations of Lifestyle Medicine*, 300.
[98] Alcohol Research Current Reviews Editorial Staff. "*Drinking Patterns and Their Definition.*"
[99] Sherzai and Sherzai, *The 30-Day Alzheimer's Solution*, part 1.

Low Risk Drinking Limits	Women	Men
On a single DAY	No more than 1 drink on any day	No more than 2 drinks on any day
	AND	AND
Per WEEK	No more than 7 drinks per week	No more than 14 drinks per week
Binge Drinking	4 or more drinks within 2-hr period	5 or more drinks within 2-hr period
Heavy Use	More than 3 on one day or more than 7 per week	More than 4 on one day or more than 14 per week

When determining your alcohol use, it is important to define what "one drink" looks like. The table below, adapted from NIH guidelines,[100] displays the fluid volume and alcohol content for typical alcoholic beverages.

12 fluid ounces of regular beer	*8–9 fluid ounces of malt liquor*	*5 fluid ounces of table wine*	*1.5 fluid ounce shot of 80-proof spirits (whiskey, gin, rum, vodka, tequila, etc.)*
About 5% alcohol	About 7% alcohol	About 12% alcohol	About 40% alcohol
The percent of "pure" alcohol, expressed here as alcohol by volume (alc/vol), varies by beverage			

You can see when thinking about your own alcohol use, it is important to not only count the number of drinks you consume but also the size and type of drink you are consuming; one of your drinks may count for two or more based on your glass size and type of alcohol. I've included a quick audit tool on the book resource website. Consult with your healthcare provider should you desire further assistance and support.

---

[100] Alcohol Research Current Reviews Editorial Staff. *"Drinking Patterns and Their Definition."*

Attribute #2 Eliminating Tobacco & Other Risky Substances

Over 15 percent of all adults are current smokers and 3 percent use smokeless tobacco products.[101] Research consistently shows us that using tobacco products is detrimental to one's health, but many individuals continue to practice this unhealthy behavior.[102] Smoking harms almost every organ in the body. Effects of smoking on health and longevity include but are not limited to:

- Risk factor for heart disease
- Damage to teeth and gums
- Risk for Type 2 Diabetes
- Risk for bladder cancer
- Weakens immune system
- Diminished skin elasticity
- Reduces muscular strength and flexibility
- Increases macular degeneration in the eyes
- Most common cause of chronic lung disease[103]

Smokers smoke fewer cigarettes than in the past, but today's smokers are at a higher risk of cancer due to changes in cigarettes—there are 70 carcinogenic chemicals in a cigarette.[104] However, people who are ready can and do quit smoking; there are more former smokers in the world now than there are current smokers. Health benefits can be experienced minutes after tobacco cessation, due to immediate physiologic effects such as a decrease in heart rate and blood pressure. After three weeks, lung function and circulation improve, after one month, coughing and wheezing decrease, and after one year, the risks for cancer, heart disease, and chronic obstructive pulmonary disease (COPD) decrease.[105] Most smokers say they want to quit; however, people are more successful with evidence-based treatments and support. Evidence-based programs can more than double successful quit rates.[106] Should you desire assistance with smoking and tobacco cessation, discuss options with your healthcare provider and call 1-800-QUIT-NOW.

Important Note *This section provides only a high-level snapshot and is not meant to replace consultation with your healthcare provider and licensed therapy provider for stress management, mental health, and risky substance use support.* After you complete the development of your *Lifestyle Wellness*

[101] American College of Lifestyle Medicine, "*Lifestyle Medicine Core Competencies Program.*" mod. TC1.
[102] American College of Lifestyle Medicine, "*Lifestyle Medicine Core Competencies Program.*" mod. TC1.
[103] American College of Lifestyle Medicine, "*Lifestyle Medicine Core Competencies Program.*" mod. TC1.
[104] American College of Lifestyle Medicine, "*Lifestyle Medicine Core Competencies Program.*" mod. TC1.
[105] American College of Lifestyle Medicine, "*Lifestyle Medicine Core Competencies Program.*" mod. TC1.
[106] American College of Lifestyle Medicine, "*Lifestyle Medicine Core Competencies Program.*" mod. TC1.

Strategic Plan, I encourage you to participate in one of my ongoing programs to support the implementation of your plan.

Strategic Wellness Activities

The strategic wellness activities in this chapter focus on developing your tactics in Section 5.0: My Lifestyle Wellness Investor Mindset Tactics & Distractions for the Destress, Connect, and Protect components so you can feel more confident you are taking control of your health destiny. It's now time for you to determine your tactics to achieve your 6-month *Interim Goals* for each component and identify your strengths-based distractions to keep engaged and enthusiastic as you move forward.

1. **Complete the *Stress Management, Positivity & Social Connections, and Risky Substance Avoidance Planning* worksheet.**

   The planning worksheet is included in your investment guide. It explains each *EBQS* in more detail and describes how to interpret and balance your *Interim Goal* percentages and choose the daily, weekly, or monthly tactics and distractions that feel authentic to you.

2. **Reconfirm your 6-month *Interim Goal* percentages and select your tactics and distractions.**

   Your tactics and distractions are what you get to use to achieve your *Interim Goals* and *Future Targets* for improved Stress Management, establishing Positivity and Social Connections, and avoiding Risky Substances. Follow the instructions in the guide. See the WLM In Practice section for examples.

3. **Update Section 5.0 in your *Lifestyle Wellness Strategic Plan.***

   Transcribe your *Future Targets* and *Interim Goals* for Stress Management, Positivity & Connections, and Risky Substance Avoidance into this section.

4. **Enter your tactics and distractions in your plan.**

   Document the initial tactics and distractions you will use to achieve your *Interim Goals* for Stress Management, Positivity & Connections, and Risky Substance Avoidance.

5. **Complete the Courage & Confidence Check.**

   How did you do with creating your tactics and distractions for these components? Do your tactics and distractions for these components reflect your courage to step out of your comfort zone and try new things? How will your distraction(s) keep you on track and motivated? You've learned about evidence-based actions to support stress management, connections & positivity, and risky substance avoidance; what makes the tactics you've chosen feel *new*, innovative, and aligned with your strengths?

WLM in Practice

Sheila decided to work toward her *Future Target* of 70 percent to improve her stress management and enhance her feelings of mental well-being. She chose not to set an *Interim Goal*. For stress adaptation and coping, her target was to achieve 70 percent of her days ($30 \times .70 = 21$ days) during the month in which she felt in control of her responsibilities, her reactions to unexpected situations, and her ability to use healthy coping strategies to manage and handle stressful personal and work issues. For increased mental well-being, her target was to achieve 70 percent of her days during the month in which she felt free from anxiety, worry, and depressed mood, and she experienced interest and pleasure in doing activities she enjoyed. Three of the tactics and distractions she chose were:

- Using birthday candle breathing after ending a stressful call with a client to calm her (tactic); then she would journal for five minutes to download and examine her thoughts instead of going to the breakroom to stress eat (distraction)
- Take daily fifteen-minute walks in nature or go to her favorite place to relax, observe her surroundings, and reconnect with her true self while listening to meditative music using a phone app (distraction)
- Scheduling two, ten-minute mindfulness breaks (tactic) throughout the day using an alarm and app on her phone (distraction)

Her *Future Target* for Positivity & Social Connections was 60 percent. She would focus on achieving 60 percent of her days ($30 \times .60 = 18$ days) during the month in which she experienced balance with the people, places, things, ideas, information, and activities that provided positive feelings of connection. To enhance her positive, possibilities mindset, she would focus on achieving 60 percent of her days in which she experienced feelings of positivity, gratefulness, and purpose. Three of the tactics she chose were:

- Practice gratefulness every morning when waiting for her tea to brew (tactic), highlighting her accomplishments from the previous day and what to look forward to today and reframing her feelings of negativity (distraction)
- Enroll in an art class (tactic) to connect with her creative side and expand her social network (distraction)
- Volunteer at a local charity she supports (tactic) to help others in need and give back (distraction)

Sheila opted for her Alcohol Avoidance *Future Target* of 30 percent, which aligns with the minimum NIH guidelines. She did not use tobacco or other substances and felt comfortable keeping her alcohol intake to one glass per day in the evening. She stayed mindful about adding the correct volume to her glass by using a measuring device to ensure the correct amount. To minimize the impact on her sleep, she timed her after-dinner cocktail to be at least three hours before her desired sleep time.

✦ ✦ ✦

Now that you've completed your planning for the six lifestyle medicine components, you should be starting to see that it really is that simple to visualize your desired health and wellness using my red-yellow-green continuum of chronic disease progression and balance your tactics and distractions to potentially give you control over your health and wellness destiny. Since I embarked on my wellness journey, investing in supporting and sustaining my authentic *Wellness Vision* has become more manageable. There have never been more health and wellness options, tools, and technologies available to help you do the same. The key is first deciding what color on the continuum feels authentic to you and then aligning your tactics and distractions accordingly. You do have a choice about what you put into your body, how you choose to spend your day, and how you frame your perspective each day. You recognize the importance of managing your stress by using healthful, constructive coping methods, including positivity and connectedness. You have control over eliminating the use of risky substances with the support of your healthcare provider and outside programs. Our bodies have the incredible ability to heal themselves when given the opportunity. It is up to you to optimize stress adaptation and well-being, cultivate positive relationships and connections, and protect your body from risky substances. By doing so, combined with healthful nutrition, efficient movement, and adequate sleep, you get to increase your investment in your health and wellness and enhance your comprehensive journey toward achieving your lasting *Wellness Vision*.

Before you move forward to the next chapter, spending a little more time on Risky Substance Avoidance, specifically alcohol use, is essential. There are a lot of conflicting opinions about the use of alcohol. Television and media promote alcohol use as synonymous with socializing, relaxing, celebrating, and what you do when feeling stressed, angry, and sad. When viewing it from a health and wellness perspective, your goal, which most people do not want to hear, should be avoidance; however, some organizations say moderation is okay. When you think about moderation related to your alcohol use, ask yourself these two questions: "Why am I using it, and, if I'm unwilling to give it up, why is that?" Do you truly need it, or has it become habitual and/or have you developed a physiological and psychological need for it? There came a time when I had to ask myself these questions.

For me, alcohol was synonymous with having a good time at dinner, parties, and clubs; it helped me overcome my shyness and awkwardness. Later, I added wine to the top of my list to de-stress after work or relieve anxiety from a stressful situation. I cut back after I met my husband, who did not drink. Over the past five years along my wellness journey, I drank alcohol rarely, only at occasional work or family gatherings—that is, until my father passed away. At first it started as one glass of wine to relieve the anxiety and stress I was feeling. Then, I began drinking multiple glasses of wine daily to manage my sadness and grief. After about two months, staring at an empty wine bottle, I asked myself the questions in the previous paragraph: 1) I was using wine to medicate my anxiety, grief, and sadness; 2) Yes, I was willing to give it up, which I have since done. The moral of my story is that we all have setbacks, and that is okay. It's how you reframe the situation and what you choose to do going forward that matters.

I had experienced a devastating loss, did what I had typically done in the past, and felt the need to do; my old, preprogrammed automatic thoughts and behaviors took over. This is not uncommon following stressful experiences. However, I have since learned and have moved forward. There is no failure here, nor is there any reason to beat myself up. Since then, I've found that research findings are mixed related to the association between any amount of alcohol consumption and cognitive decline in older age. I've chosen to be on the cautious side of the research and stay aligned with my *Future Target* of 100%. I choose brain health over alcohol any day! The choice is truly up to you, however. I find many clients struggle in this area and choose to stay within the standard guidelines. Should you desire assistance with managing alcohol or substance use, be sure to talk to your healthcare provider. There are many programs and organizations available to support you as well.

By integrating tactics into your current lifestyle that align with your strengths and using distractions and support resources, you will be able to enjoy and sustain the changes you make in all six lifestyle medicine components. You are just starting your journey; eventually, you will want to invest in more healthy lifestyle choices to move you further toward your *Wellness Vision*—the green side of the chronic disease progression continuum demonstrating that you value your health as an important wealth.

You have two more critical lifestyle wellness components to explore that will impact your success, regardless of how much you are willing to invest: your *Home and Work Environments*. You get to set up your environments to support you and help you make health and wellness your easy, default choice so that you achieve your *Wellness Vision*. This is where creativity comes into play, along with your willingness to deviate from mainstream expectations about your home and work environments; you must choose "Wellness Nonconformity," which I will cover in the next chapter.

Dr. Lori's Insights

- Don't discount the importance of managing stress for great health and wellness. Identify your stress triggers and develop creative tactics and distractions to manage how you respond and adapt to stress.

- Read the book *Positivity* by Barbara Fredrickson to become more familiar with the benefits of positivity on your health and well-being and how to manage the negativity at home and work.
- Use of risky substances to relieve stress introduces more stress on the body. Don't add insult to injury. Think about other ways to protect and destress your body. It is the only one you have, so choose wisely.

CHAPTER SIXTEEN

Your Lifestyle Wellness Roadmap– Support & Thrive

Congratulations! You've identified creative and innovative tactics and distractions in all six life-style medicine components to get you started on your wellness journey. Remember, you are developing the first version of your *Lifestyle Wellness Strategic Plan*. Your plan is a living, breathing document. As you achieve your 6-month *Interim Goals*, experiment with new wellness tactics and distractions, leverage your strengths, and learn more about yourself and what feels authentic for you. Update your plan accordingly. This chapter focuses on how to optimize your home and work environments and structure your days for minimizing obstacles, so you get to make the changes that support your *Wellness Vision* and achieve your best possible self. Making changes in your environments is sometimes more challenging because you may not have control of your environment at work or at home, and you have family members and coworkers to consider. Using your growth mindset, view both as energetic challenges to transform into a *Wellness Nonconformist* in an unhealthy, conformist world. What does being a Wellness Nonconformist mean and look like? Throughout my life, I always felt different, as though I didn't fit in at home, school, or work.

I thought it was because of my personality, which I came to learn aligned more with being a studious introvert—someone more energized by books, creativity, and data versus people and connections. My family always questioned what I was doing and how I chose to live my life. I often heard the rhetorical questions, "Now what are you up to? Another degree? Will you ever settle down?" Without realizing it, I was living the life of a *nonconformist* in many ways; I was being judged using other peoples' mainstream conformist expectations. However, I didn't comprehend the magnitude until I began my lifestyle wellness journey.

If you don't realize it by now, to transform your Well-Leader Mindset™, you must have the courage and confidence to embrace *Wellness Nonconformity*. Thus far, you've decided on how much you are willing to invest to achieve your *Future Targets*. The *Wellness Nonconformity* comes into play during the implementation, that's where the challenges occur. Implementing your plan often goes against the standard American lifestyle (SAL). SAL does not promote/support extraordinary health and wellness. One of my favorite quotes from author Tommy Newberry is, "If you want to lead an extraordinary life, find out what the ordinary do—and don't do it." This applies to your health and wellness. If you want to achieve the extraordinary health and wellness you desire, you've got to go against the grain—overcome short-term, instant gratification, mainstream thinking, and external "should" pressures; that's what defending your *Wellness Nonconformity* looks like. Making supportive changes in your home and work environments will soften the mainstream and external pressures; however, making the choice to set up your environments to support extraordinary health and wellness means choosing to become a *Wellness Nonconformist*, someone who:

- chooses the road less traveled,
- chooses to stand out from mainstream pressures, and
- chooses to often feel awkward and out of place in an unhealthy world!

Stepping out of the routine of an unhealthy world means you get to set up your life and your environments in a way to retire old comfortable habits and routines and replace them with new ones that better fit your desire for a health-promoting life (which, BTW, may be less popular with friends and family, and even you at first). Even though you know it is the right thing to do, it may take some time for you to transition and accept a change as your new healthy normal (Use the positive transition process and losing→gaining activity to help with your transition.). Take a few minutes to think about the areas and situations in your home and work environments that you know don't support extraordinary health and wellness. How easy or difficult will it be for you to make changes? Do you have control, or will you need to gather the support of others? What challenges and obstacles will you encounter? Just like you learned with the six lifestyle wellness components, you may decide to set *Interim Goals* for the changes to your home and work environments to allow time for you and others to transition.

Your goal is to set up your home and work environments in ways that make the healthier choices the most convenient, attractive, and commonplace, and make the least healthy choices inconvenient and hidden. Doing so allows you to rely *less* on your willpower. Willpower is fragile and limited, but mindless habits can last forever. You will be more successful in making the changes in all the lifestyle wellness components when you integrate them into your life, so they become "healthy mindless habits" as quickly as possible. Creating supportive environments can do just that; becoming healthy and well by designing your work and home environments works better than using willpower.[107] It's sometimes easier to change your environment to support and thrive throughout your wellness journey than to change your mind. Willpower alone won't conquer bad habits for 90 percent of people.[108] No matter how healthy your intentions, when confronted with a long-enough stream of pressures, frustrations, and temptations, eventually you may cave and take the path of least resistance.

Supportive Home Environment

The *Evidence-Based Quality Standard* for this component is:

- Optimize and design your home life to support wellness by *making healthy choices the default* and *prioritizing self-care.*

Chronic Disease Progression Potential	Incite & Accelerate (red)		Slow (orange)		Mitigate & Arrest (yellow)		Prevent & Reverse (green)		
Supportive Home Environment *EBQS:*	Unsupportive Home Life					Supportive Home Life			
Rating Range (%)	10	20	30	40	50	60	70	80	90	100

Think about your home environment—not only the physical layout, room locations, furniture, and outside space, but how you "live" at home. Just as organizations have a culture, your home life has a culture; is it more of a sedentary, unhealthy culture, or that of an active, health-oriented culture? Is your living room more of a sedentary-living room or a well-living room? Is your kitchen rarely used, or is it an experimental haven for creative, whole food, plant-based cooking? Is your pantry stocked with processed, unhealthy food-like items, or do you see a rainbow of whole plant foods? Does your

---

[107] Wansink, *Slim by Design*, intro.
[108] Wansink, *Slim by Design*, intro.

family hide out in their own spaces, or do they collaborate and actively engage together? Are you left to manage everything at home on your own, or do you have the support of other family members? Does your home motivate you to head straight for the couch after work, or does it invite a calm, relaxing experience for you to reenergize? These are all components that make up your home culture. Does your current home culture have the potential to enhance (10), somewhat support (5), or detract from (1) the health and wellness you desire?

Your goal for reimagining your home environment is creating a home culture that works with you every day, including supporting your health and wellness, fueling your workouts with nutritious foods, maintaining safety and security, and encouraging your relaxation and recovery.[109] Once you make the right changes to your home environment, you get to engage in healthier behaviors without thinking about it. You make healthy decisions even when you've had a tough day at work and your brain is stressed, tired, or on autopilot.

WLM in Practice

The following client examples illustrate how each change in home environment impacts the six lifestyle medicine components: Eat (E), Movement (M), Sleep (S), Destress (D), Avoidance of Risky Substances (A), and Positivity & Connections (C). Haley and her husband redesigned their kitchen, eating areas, and food choice options. They made healthier foods more visible and accessible on the counter; cleaned out the junk from the pantry; and made it easier to enjoy plant-based meals by using a meal-delivery service three times per week. Her husband does the cooking and they eat together as much as possible. They plan time each week to create individual portions for snacks and have established a fresh food prep day together during which they discuss the book they are reading to engage them and make preparing for healthy eating enjoyable (E,S,D,C).

Sheila created a Do-Not-Disturb, My-Time Wellness Space. She set up a section of her bedroom as her personal wellness space where she can relax and rejuvenate instead of drinking wine. She spends ten-to-fifteen minutes there after work in the evening or whenever she needs to destress. Her husband and children know to stay away when she is in her space (M,S,D,A,C).

Marjorie created her *well-living* room. She blew off the cobwebs from her treadmill and moved it to her living room from the basement and rearranged her furniture to create an area for stretching and yoga. She uses her treadmill for a ten-to-twenty-minute moderate intensity cardio session to rejuvenate, walk during a meeting, read her favorite book or news feed, or catch up on a streaming episode. Marjorie's friend, a seamstress, created a cover for her treadmill when folded and not in use

---

[109] Gold, *Wellness by Design*, intro.

that matched the décor of her living room (M,S,D,C).

An important home environmental consideration I want to touch on before you move on is the use of and exposure to chemicals and carcinogens in cleaning products, air fresheners, skin and personal care products, makeup, plastics, tap water, lawn and pest care products, etc. When I started my journey, there were not many alternatives available. Now you can find numerous plant-based, vegan, and nontoxic options for all of these. A big one for me was how to keep my dog safe; that's where I started. Research supports that synthetic air fresheners, carpet and floor cleaners, laundry detergents, and other toxic chemicals are linked to cancer and other neurological issues in dogs.[110] I changed my air fresheners to essential oils and purchased plant-based, nontoxic options for all my cleaning products. The Environmental Working Group provides a website and product lists for cleaning and personal care products. You can review a full list of EWG verified products with grades for all the ingredients.[111] Before I purchase any product, I check the EWG product lists and review the ingredients. The good news is that plant-based, nontoxic cleaning and personal care items are readily available in big box stores, most grocery stores, and online.

Supportive Work Environment

The *Evidence-Based Quality Standard* for this component is:

- Optimize and design your work life to *elevate support for wellness at work* and integrate and engage in *self-care throughout the workday.*

Chronic Disease Progression Potential	Incite & Accelerate (red)			Slow (orange)		Mitigate & Arrest (yellow)			Prevent & Reverse (green)	
Supportive Work Environment *EBQS*:	Unsupportive Work Life							Supportive Work Life		
Rating Range (%)	10	20	30	40	50	60	70	80	90	100

Now, it's time to think about your work environment—your primary office location, home office,

---

[110] Becker and Habib, *The Forever Dog.* chap 10.
[111] Environmental Working Group. *"EWG Verified™."*

or mobile office if you travel. Research supports that work is the number one cause of stress, which is a big driver of chronic disease; the rise of chronic disease and associated costs have a direct impact on business and employee well-being.[112] You most likely spend at least one-third of your day or more at work, not including getting ready and commuting time. Is your primary work location a place that embodies health and wellness? If you work from home, does your home office provide a comfortable, stress-free environment for you to engage and feel productive? If you work for a medium to large organization, you may have an employee wellness program; most small organizations offer some level of wellness benefits or incentives as well. Are you taking advantage of those? What is the wellness culture of your organization? Is it okay to take ten minutes to rejuvenate, are healthy meal options available, and are long work hours the exception not the rule?

You may not have control over making changes to your work environment. As a leader, you do have control over your attitude and how you structure your workday and interactions. Similar to your home environment, when you restructure your workspace and workday, you'll exercise your *Wellness Nonconformity* by defending and making healthier choices your default. You get to make healthy decisions even when swamped at work with back-to-back meetings and a never-ending to-do list. What other choice do you have?

The importance of recognizing how your home and work environments and societal norms continually impact and try to derail all areas of your wellness journey is critically important and something that is often overlooked. It's time to step back and examine how your environments support your unhealthy default reality—those automatic, everyday thoughts and behaviors you aren't sure why you keep thinking and doing without questioning the impact they have on your life. Making healthy choices requires steering around a slew of well-established social norms and widely accepted expectations. In other words, it requires you to dare to be the *Wellness Nonconformist*, to be different from society's prevailing norms and conventions, which is not always easy! Fortunately, there are a lot of small, innovative, adventurous, and proven solutions from behavioral economics and psychology that will help you become well by design. Wellness by design is about deliberately changing all your environments so that you, your family, and even your coworkers are affected by *your* wellness. You see the simple actions you can take to achieve your wellness goals without really having to work harder at it, and you can get others to help and support you and even join in.

---

[112] Miller, Williams, and O'Neill. *The Healthy Workplace Nudge*, chap 1.

WLM in Practice

The following client examples illustrate how each work environment change impacts the six lifestyle medicine components: Eat (E), Movement (M), Sleep (S), Destress (D), Avoidance of Risky Substances (A), and Positivity & Connections (C). Marnie transformed into a healthy squirrel at work. She learned that research supports that people who have candy in or on their desks weigh on average 15.4 pounds more than those who do not. She eliminated all the snacks in her desk and switched to healthier choices to start a new tradition (E,S,D). Also, Marnie "amped up" her workday. She used the *Compendium of Activities* list you reviewed in the Movement section to amplify her daily work activities to increase her METs. She ordered a standing desk (1.8 METs), got a headset so she could walk while on the phone (2.0 METs), and held walking meetings (2.5 METs) when appropriate (M,S,D,C).

Haley chose to minimize certain activities that enabled unhealthy behaviors, such as going out for drinks after work. She realized that people in some of her work social circles were affecting her healthy behavior choices. She decided to spend less time with them and find ways to leverage the three degrees of separation rule: hang out with healthy people who hang out with healthy people who hang out with healthy people, and so on (E,M,S,D,A,C).

Marjorie chose to take the long way at work by adding a little extra distance and movement to her workday. She parked further away and on the top level of the parking garage to take the stairs. She added an extra lap or more around the office area when she used the restroom and filled her water bottle (E,M,S,D).

Strategic Wellness Activities

The strategic wellness activities in this chapter focus on how to optimize your home and work environments and structure your days to integrate and elevate daily lifestyle wellness tactics and distractions and minimize obstacles, so you can make the changes you desire to support your *Wellness Vision* and achieve your best possible self. You will document your tactics and distractions for structuring your home and work environments so you can feel more confident you can easily implement your *Lifestyle Wellness Strategic Plan* at home and work and take control of your health destiny. It's now time for you to determine your tactics to achieve your 6-month *Interim Goals* for each environment and identify your strengths-based distractions to keep engaged and enthusiastic as you move forward.

1. **Complete the *Supportive Environments Planning* worksheet.**

   The planning worksheet is included in your investment guide. It explains each *EBQS* in more detail and describes how to interpret and balance your *Interim Goal* percentages and choose the daily, weekly, or monthly tactics and distractions that feel authentic to you.

2. **Reconfirm your 6-month *Interim Goal* percentages and select your tactics and distractions.**

   Your tactics and distractions are what you get to use to achieve your *Interim Goals* and *Future Targets* for creating Supportive Home & Work Environments. Follow the instructions in the guide. See the WLM In Practice section for examples.

3. **Complete Section 5.1 My Lifestyle Wellness by Design in your *Lifestyle Wellness Strategic Plan.***

   Transcribe your *Future Targets* and *Interim Goals* for Supportive Home & Work Environments and the initial tactics and distractions you will use to achieve these goals and targets.

4. **Conduct a final review of Sections 5.0 and 5.1 in your plan.**

   These sections should be complete. For all eight lifestyle wellness components, confirm that you have entered all your *Interim Goals*, *Future Targets*, and the tactics and distractions you are willing to invest in over the next six months. Make adjustments to ensure your tactics and distractions feel authentic to you.

5. **Complete the Courage & Confidence Check.**

   How did you do with creating your tactics and distractions for creating supportive environments at home and work? How do your tactics and distractions reflect your courage to make the changes you desire to make, involve your family and coworkers, and try new things? Aligning your tactics and distractions for creating supportive home and work environments with your strengths will increase your confidence in your ability to make the changes to support your lifelong health and wellness journey.

As I wrote at the start of this chapter, I was a *Wellness Nonconformist* in an unhealthy conformist world long before I realized it. My husband and I have always had a dedicated workout room with all the equipment we desired. I reorganized my kitchen and pantry to highlight healthy snacks and have all the gadgets to make whole food, plant-based meals. My office setup supports incorporating movement throughout my day and during work meetings. I set up a mindfulness spot that my husband knows to stay away from when I am there, and I've optimized my sleep environment and routine to achieve consistent quality. Finally, I worked with a mindset coach to develop my possibilities thinking and manage stressful home and work situations, and I've eliminated the use of risky substances—I thought I had everything covered.

After my father passed away in January 2021, I hit a health and wellness brick wall. The changes I made were no longer supporting me. I struggled with my health and wellness for about six months, primarily with movement and drinking wine daily. Eventually, I was able to refocus my tactics and distractions to get all components back on track, except for the movement component. The expansive workout room in our dark basement that we had enjoyed for the past three years wasn't going to cut it any longer. I couldn't find the motivation to go to that dark place. I knew I needed something new, bright, sunny, and more "in my face" to motivate me. I wanted wellness to be the center of my life again. I called upon my Wellness Nonconformity to transform my conventional sedentary-living room—the largest, brightest, most central room in the house and one that we rarely used—into my well-living room. Success! I experienced the incredible power of stepping out of mainstream conventions. Movement is more accessible and convenient. I use the room as my second office for my morning creativity and mindfulness sessions on my WaterRower® and treadmill desk webinars and meetings when I decide to walk instead of using the standing desk in my office.

As a family, we now enjoy gathering in our new well-living room to have fun and create healthy moments together. This was one of the most energizing changes I've ever experienced. I still do have a cozy, small sedentary-living room, in a spare bedroom where we watch movies on Saturday or Sunday. Sometimes it takes bold changes to your home and work environments to jumpstart your wellness and make it central to your life. You will optimize your health and wellness investment when your *Lifestyle Wellness Strategic Plan* incorporates vital changes to your home and work environments— changes that make your new lifestyle wellness tactics and distractions easy and automatic!

Changing your home and work environments helps you think more strategically and long-term about your health and wellness—you create the structure and conditions on purpose that support living your *Wellness Vision* every day. When you don't create wellness-supportive environments, you fail to see the forest for the trees by focusing only on the details, not the big picture. Developing your *Lifestyle Wellness Strategic Plan* ensures you take the time to envision the forest (environments) and the trees (tactics and distractions). As a result, you understand the complete long-term picture and have the information to make informed decisions about your health and wellness investments. You choose to become a strategic health seeker by treating your health as an important wealth. However, this does not simply happen on its own. By making changes in your thinking and environment, healthy behaviors become the norm, and you exert minimal willpower. Your ringing phone, endless texts and emails, undone to-do list, and your kids will still be there. You can manage all these things better, with less stress, when your life has been set up strategically to be *well-by-design*. Even the smartest, most disciplined, health-conscious fanatics can be easily influenced by their surroundings, even when they know it is happening. The key is recognizing when this is happening. Then invoke the practices, tactics, and distractions you developed to continue living the *Wellness Vision* you constructed in your *Lifestyle Wellness Strategic Plan*!

Dr. Lori's Insights

- Changes in your work and home environments are required to successfully implement your *Lifestyle Wellness Strategic Plan.* Don't discount the importance of supportive environments to help you make healthier choices without having to think about it, and engage significant others at home and coworkers to support your wellness journey.
- Structure your home and work environments and lifestyle in a way that does not deplete your willpower; make healthy behaviors automatic using *in your face* changes.
- Identify changes you can make to your home and work environments that will support your health goals without creating much additional effort on your part. You may have to *educate* others and let them know how to support you.
- Experiment with changes to see what works for you and give the change a chance to work. If it is not working for you after two weeks, try something new. Experimenting is the essence of a growth mindset and a long-term, savvy health and wellness investor.

CHAPTER SEVENTEEN

Your Lifestyle Wellness Index— Optimize Your Investment

The previous three chapters were packed with evidence-based standards, recommendations, and resources to create thoughtful tactics and distractions that align with your belief that you can and you will achieve your *Wellness Vision*—actions that inspire you to invest in and sustain your authentic health and wellness journey. You may be feeling a bit overwhelmed and exhausted; this is normal. As with typical strategic planning in your business, planning your lifestyle wellness is no less exhausting and it takes just as much—or more—brain power and focused effort.

Learning about the components of lifestyle wellness and creating your own innovative tactics for each component aligned with your strengths while designing your environments to make wellness automatic will set you up for success this time. Knowing that you potentially have control over the progression, reversal, and prevention of chronic diseases of lifestyle by simply changing your behaviors elevates your energy and motivation. You may *no longer* be at the mercy of your genetics. You *can, and you will* change your destiny. It's about how much you are willing to invest to potentially live a long, healthy, disease-free lifestyle. You choose to do so by mindfully integrating lifestyle wellness into everything you do and then sticking with it, fine-tuning what works for you, and creating new behavior patterns that feel genuine and effortless—that's authentic wellness.

When I learned that I had the power to influence my health and wellness destiny, I jumped all in and never looked back; who knew I could have such control? I'm not really a control freak, contrary to what my five sisters think. I have shifted my perspective and reframed this as me defending my health and wellness destiny by exerting my growth and possibilities mindset—exercising my strategic and future-oriented wellness investment mindset. It's time to take a moment to pause, catch your breath, and embrace the tactics and distractions you get to implement to guide your forward progression. Do your tactics reflect that you have shifted toward a growth, long-term investor mindset? How far do you see yourself going into the future to influence your health and wellness destiny? Are you ready to go full speed or dial it back and make a slower transformation? You decide; it must feel authentic to you.

If you are still a bit unsure, this may be a great time for a *Wellness Strategy Session* to review your *Lifestyle Wellness Strategic Plan* thus far, clear any final roadblocks, and shift your mindset to one that energizes and focuses you on your future possibilities. The link to schedule your *Wellness Strategy Session* with me is located on the book resource website. If you believe Sections 5.0 and 5.1 of your plan are at least 80 percent, you are ready to move forward. You have clarity on your *Future Targets*, 6-month *Interim Goals*, and tactics and distractions. This is *how* you've decided to begin your journey to creating a life that reflects the best version of yourself. You believe your *Interim Goals* are achievable within the six-month planning horizon. You believe the tactics to achieve your *Interim Goals* reflect a chain reaction of bridge beliefs that line up to move you closer toward the lifestyle wellness *Future Targets* you've determined will provide positive benefits throughout your life. You're confident the strengths-based distractions you added will make the tactics more engaging and enjoyable for you and not elicit the "ugh" feeling about a tactic. *Ugh-tactics* won't stick in the long term. To avoid the *ugh* factor, the best strategy is to incorporate small new habits throughout the day that don't require much effort yet have a powerful compounding effect if you repeat them often enough.

In the final chapters, you complete the remaining sections of your *Lifestyle Wellness Strategic Plan* that support and sustain your confidence and readiness. These sections are the critical last pieces of the puzzle. They focus on monitoring and accountability to keep you on track and building resilience using contingencies when life and your brain get in the way. You know even the best laid plans are *always* subject to change; the same is true for your *Lifestyle Wellness Strategic Plan*.

Think of your final plan as simply the *starting point* for your wellness journey. When you begin implementing your tactics to achieve the *Evidence-Based Quality Standards* for all lifestyle wellness components, you are experimenting with the tactics and distractions you've chosen that align with your strengths that will help you achieve the goals you've set forth. As with any plan, even in business, you want to know if your plan is consistently working for you after you've implemented it. Are you achieving the value and return on your *wellness investment*? Are you making progress toward achieving your lifestyle wellness *Future Targets*?

Health is a priceless wealth. I can't say it enough because I get to experience it now and will consistently defend my "Whealth." How will you know if you are optimizing your investment in your lifelong health and wellness? By treating your lifestyle wellness journey more like you do your wealth, by investing in your *Wellness Vision* for the long term, and by valuing your health while you are gaining it, not just focusing on it after you lose it. If we treated our lifestyle wellness like we do our wealth, we would make it a priority, work hard to pass on our wellness legacy to our children, put in the extra effort today to achieve a greater return later, and young people would aspire to it.[113] Based on what is promoted as the standard American lifestyle, the availability of endless junk food options, and all the get-fit and get-healthy-quick solutions that eventually lead back to *health and wellness bankruptcy*, this is not the case.

I admit that I did not treat my health as important as wealth until I began my lifestyle wellness journey five years ago. I was a health-conscious person, but I invested more time and effort in the health of my education, career, family, and financial status. When one of those areas became challenging or required more effort, my health and wellness always fell to the bottom of the list. The thing I didn't realize back then was that I didn't have to make a trade-off or choose. The same is true for you; you get to have it all! And you decide what *it all* looks like. Who wants to reach retirement age well-educated with a fulfilling career and well off financially but in poor health, unable to enjoy retirement and beyond? You see now that it doesn't have to be this way. You can, and you will change this.

Our society makes it clear that responsible adults take care of their money but provides no such guidance for those who neglect their health. However, health is not like wealth; it is vastly *more important*. Just ask someone who has one but not the other.[114] Creating and implementing your *Lifestyle Wellness Strategic Plan* elevates your health and wellness to a higher level of wealth by making it a strategic priority to live your best life for the rest of your life. It becomes your health and wellness retirement strategy, but you benefit from it *now*; there are no penalties for early withdrawal, and it's tax free, no 1099-R to file. Your *Lifestyle Wellness Strategic Plan* helps you shift your mindset to one that believes in and values investment in your health for the long term. It helps you step out of the 30-, 60-, or 90 day get-fit (rich)-quick mentality.

Because you are treating your health and wellness as a long-term, health-is-a-priceless-wealth investment strategy, traditional tracking and progress measurement processes won't work. Who wants to count calories, steps, glasses of water consumed, food composition, hours of quality time with your children, etc., for the rest of your life? Not me! When I started my strategic journey, I knew I had to track things a bit closer for a few months after I implemented my plan; however, now

---

[113] Katz, "*What if Health Were More Like Wealth?*"
[114] Katz, "*What if Health Were More Like Wealth?*"

I just "Do," with minimal tracking. I eat, move, sleep, destress, connect, and protect my health by applying the tactics and distractions I've chosen and have integrated seamlessly into my life. I've set up my home and work environments so I can effortlessly live the lifestyle of wellness I created for myself. I make my *Wellness Vision* a reality every day, and it feels authentic and effortless! It all starts with creating a plan that fits your life. Living your authentic *Lifestyle Wellness Strategic Plan* is the antidote—you get to neutralize your wellness cognitive dissonance.

Remember, when you take a strategic approach to wellness, you are focused on the forest, not the individual trees. Think about this related to your long-term financial investments; do you check the performance of your 401k or retirement accounts every hour, every day, or every week? You may feel confident in your investment portfolio and simply review your monthly or quarterly statements. You've chosen the funds you want to invest in, the level of risk you want to accept, and you let your investments perform; is this starting to sound familiar? You've prioritized the lifestyle wellness components, chosen the level of chronic disease progression risk you want to accept, and you've decided on the tactics and distractions. All that is left is for *you* to perform and then evaluate your progress using your weekly, monthly, or quarterly health and wellness investment statements.

Your Lifestyle Wellness Index (LWI) Measurement Plan

I created the *Lifestyle Wellness Index* to help you begin viewing your *Lifestyle Wellness Strategic Plan* to achieve your *Wellness Vision* as a strategic, long-term investment and retirement (and beyond) strategy that you get to benefit from now and every day along the way. You most likely have a 401(k) and/or other retirement investment accounts. Think of your *LWI* as your health and wellness index fund or ETF (exchange-traded fund) that tracks the performance of a specific benchmark or *index*. In this case, your benchmarks are the *Evidence-Based Quality Standards* for the eight lifestyle wellness components in your *health and wellness portfolio*. You've set your desired *Future Targets* and 6-month *Interim Goals*, which represent the level of potential chronic disease progression risk (return) you choose to accept for each—just like you would for your financial investments. Unlike a financial index fund, however, you are your *fund manager* and get to choose the tactics and distractions (individual stocks) you want in each component of your portfolio.

As you implement your *Lifestyle Wellness Strategic Plan*, you decide how often you want to evaluate how you are progressing toward the 6-month *Interim Goals* and *Future Targets* you've set that align with your *Wellness Vision*. At each measurement point, you examine the alignment between your performance and how you are tracking toward achieving your goals and targets. It doesn't matter if your performance was lower than planned today, yesterday, or last week; it's about what happens in the long term, just like with your long-term retirement investments. Even if your performance seems lower than planned, as long as you are taking action, you are still making progress toward your long-term *Future Target*. Similar to a long-term investment, your *LWI* keeps you focused on what ultimately matters—transforming your mindset to one of growth and possibilities by staying focused not on the trees but the forest—your *Wellness Vision*. You are confident the tactics you have chosen are giving you the highest probability that your cumulative, evidence-based actions are potentially adding years to your life and life to your years. As the fund manager, you will most likely adjust your *stock picks* (tactics and distractions) based on what the *market* (your life situation) will bear; you will be choosing, experimenting, and trading stocks in your *LWI* portfolio for the rest of your life. The *Evidence-Based Quality Standards* don't change, but you may decide to adjust your chronic disease progression risk acceptance by choosing to do more and adding new aligned tactics and distractions to your lifestyle wellness portfolio.

Even though you are looking strategically, you still must track and monitor your tactics and distractions at some level, which is always up to you. I suggest weekly monitoring overall, but you should use a method to quickly make a note about daily performance, at least in the short term. Some of my clients have used journals, smartwatches, fitness and nutrition apps, calendar appointments and tasks, or a whiteboard. You get to decide what works for you to track the effectiveness of the tactics and distractions you've chosen to achieve your 6-month *Interim Goals* for each lifestyle component. Keep them quick, basic, and high-level—something you can consistently commit to doing.

Just as you are experimenting with your tactics and distractions, try different measurement methods for each lifestyle wellness component. Your long-term measurement goal is to just do; work your plan with minimal effort for measurement. You will get there. For your *LWI* performance evaluation, I recommend evaluating components weekly for the first two-to-three months after implementing your *Lifestyle Wellness Strategic Plan*. During the first few months, you are experimenting, reviewing lessons learned, transforming your mindset, and most likely adjusting the *stocks in your portfolio* (tactics and distractions) until you find what you can comfortably perform and what fits and feels authentic to you. Eventually, you won't have to track your tactics any longer, and your *subconscious healthy mindset* will take over. Acting in healthy ways integrated throughout your day has become what you do and what you like to do; it feels right without having to think about it.

As I implemented my own *Lifestyle Wellness Strategic Plan*, I found that a typical, short-term feedback and measurement process that focused on tactics and short-term measures such as weight loss, daily steps, food logs, or lab tests wouldn't work for me. I'm not an app person, and I didn't want to spend time tracking the minutia. I had crafted my strategy, set my *Interim Goals* and *Future Targets*, and aligned my tactics and distractions. I knew what to do, so I focused on the *doing* by implementing my strategic plan and making the *doing* work for me throughout my day. I was tired of beating myself up like I had done in the past when I didn't quite achieve my goals that day or week. Even though I didn't fully achieve my goals, I was still making progress, learning about myself, and transforming my mindset, which definitely matters! Unfortunately, you may be so used to SMART goals and typical health and wellness measurement processes that focus on deficiencies, abnormalities, limitations, and gaps in what you didn't accomplish—the impacts of your past. What a downer and a recipe for self-loathing that is! You've already spent too much time in this world focusing and ruminating on your past and what you see in the daily news—things you can't change. Instead, it's time to focus on the experiences and possibilities your health and wellness investments will bring to your future.

When it comes to your health and wellness, your past is your past and *does not* have to equal your future. Your failures do not define you; you get to use them to lead you to more amazing future possibilities. That's the purpose of your *LWI* performance evaluation. It is future-oriented and focuses on what you can control by helping you overpower your emotions and highlighting taking action *and* sometimes failing! A growth mindset seeks out challenges and failures. It's okay to try things and fail; that means you are putting yourself out there by experimenting and creating opportunities to grow your health and wellness investments. You are finding what will work for you. Effectively diversifying and managing the *stocks* in your *LWI* will pay short-term dividends, long-term dividends, and then some by potentially adding life to your years and years to your life! It's been five years for me, and my *LWI* portfolio is on its way toward achieving my future performance expectations well before retirement and beyond; I've already achieved amazing health and wellness for *someone my age*. As my personal health and wellness fund manager, I focus on achieving optimum results for the level of input that feels authentic to me. As of this writing, my

LWI portfolio is consistently performing at the following levels:

LWI Component	Current Monthly Performance	Future Target
Nutrition	95%	100%
Movement	90%	100%
Sleep	80%	90%
Stress Management	75%	90%
Connections & Positivity	80%	100%
Risky Substance Avoidance	100%	100%
Supportive Home Environment	90%	90%
Supportive Work Environment	80%	90%
Overall LWI Average Performance	**86.25%**	**95%**

Just like my financial investments, my *LWI* portfolio performance often fluctuates daily and may change based on new situations and issues that arise. I don't focus on the daily fluctuations— that would make me crazy! I've honed the tactics and distractions I use over the years and stay in continuous improvement mode. I know what to do to consistently achieve long-term high performance internally (mindset, mental well-being, and body systems functioning) and externally (body composition, strength, agility, and pain-free mobility and functionality) despite the setbacks and normal *market* (life) fluctuations. My sleep quality will always be a work in progress as well as building my possibilities mindset and stress management capabilities. I've structured my home and work environments to be extremely supportive; however, normal, and sometimes unexpected, family obligations—I'm also a caregiver for my 90-year-old mother who lives in an adjacent inlaw apartment in my home—require me to be a bit more flexible and adapt my plan to fit the situation. I can still maintain my healthy behaviors but initiate my resilience tactics (you will work on this in the next chapter) to keep my *LWI* portfolio progressing toward my ultimate *Wellness Vision*.

Your *LWI* gives you the information to decide what to do next and how to be an effective fund manager for the wealth of your health. You will gauge how you are feeling about the effectiveness of your tactics and distractions and determine whether you are making progress toward your *Wellness Vision* and you may decide to change direction or feel ready to increase your investment. Your *LWI* gives you the information to decide what to do next, how to be an effective fund manager for the wealth of your health. Think about your business—if you didn't have metrics and measurements, you wouldn't know how your business was doing or when to change course. Setting up your basic measurement process will help you decide if you want to do more, scale back, make changes to your plan, or focus more on another lifestyle wellness component. Your *Lifestyle Wellness Index* keeps you focused not on your health and wellness reality but on becoming a savvy wellness investment fund manager; who knew? This is all part of your Well-Leader Mindset™ strategic progression and your forward focus on creating your best self now and into the future.

Strategic Wellness Activities

The strategic wellness activities in this chapter help you create a measurement plan that includes some basic techniques to measure the implementation and effectiveness of your tactics and distractions and the frequency of measurement—you decide what works for you. You also get to accept the challenge of becoming your *Lifestyle Wellness Index* fund manager to evaluate and balance the ongoing effectiveness of your *Lifestyle Wellness Strategic Plan* through periodic review and evaluation. As noted earlier, to evaluate your *LWI*, I recommend weekly reviews for the first two-to-three months so you can reflect, learn, and adapt your tactics, distractions, and tracking processes. You most likely do this already with the new financial investments you make—monitor the investment more closely at first and then scale back your monitoring. Also, during the first few months of implementing your plan, you may decide to do more to potentially reduce your chronic disease development risk by moving your goals and targets further toward the green range of the continuum.

1. **Complete the *Lifestyle Wellness Index (LWI) Measurement* worksheet.**

   The measurement worksheet in your investment guide helps you you decide the investment tracking and monitoring process that works best for you. Follow the instructions and process in the guide to complete the worksheet.

2. **Complete Section 6.0 My Lifestyle Wellness Index (LWI) Measurement Plan in your *Lifestyle Wellness Strategic Plan*.**

   Transcribe your measurement tactics and frequency to monitor and maintain your awareness of how you are doing for each component. Your measurements should provide enough information for you to decide if you want to adjust your tactics and distractions to achieve and sustain your long-term wellness transformation.

3. **Download the *LWI Statement Tracking* template.**

   Access the spreadsheet template on the book resource website. I've created this spreadsheet for you to monitor your plan performance easily and prepare your weekly, monthly, and quarterly *LWI Statements*. Follow the instructions in the guide to setup your spreadsheet.

4. **Complete the Courage & Confidence Check.**

   How did you do with creating your measurement plan and preparing yourself to take on your new role of fund manager for your *Lifestyle Wellness Index*? Do your measurement practices reflect your courage to maintain a long-term, neutral, and intentional perspective when it comes to evaluating your progress toward optimizing your investment in your health and wellness? This means you don't go negative—all progress is good. Lifestyle medicine is about making confident, consistent, forward progress, weathering the ups and downs, and using your *LWI* measurement plan to identify when you may need to adjust your focus to stay on track with your *Wellness Vision*.

Your *LWI* evaluations focus more on your evolving wellness investor mindset and less on the tactics; however, you will still enter your alignment with your *Interim Goals* and *Future Targets* each measurement period. I've added a qualitative component you get to use to evaluate your evolving Well-Leader Mindset™ applying the following rating scale:

E1	Emerging	Your wellness mindset is taking shape and becoming more established; you are ready to move away from your old, unhealthy reality.
E2	Envisioning	You are visualizing and imagining your wellness future as possible; you are beginning to experience the power of what is possible for you.
E3	Engaging	You are involved and connected to your strategic wellness, excited about your transformation, and committed to continue.
E4	Empowering	You are feeling courageous and confident in controlling your life and claiming and defending the health and wellness you desire.
E5	Embodying	You are experiencing the tangible benefits of your efforts; your wellness has become integrated into the thread of your being—you believe it's who you are.

Your evolving mindset matters more than how many steps you've walked, how many pounds you've lost, how many workouts you've done, or how many glasses of water you've consumed. Your Well-Leader Mindset™ is what propels you into the future and makes achieving your *Wellness Vision* (and other things) possible. When you think and believe differently, you will *be* different. You keep your beliefs ahead of where you are and leave fear and failure in the past. The performance you are expecting will come and feel natural when you get—and sustain—your Well-Leader Mindset™ right first!

WLM in Practice

Haley uses her smartwatch to align the sleep periods measured by her watch with the three *EBQS* quality sleep attributes. She focused her tactics on reducing light-sleep periods and periods of wakefulness. She documents her quality measures for all components in a daily journal she had been using prior to developing her *Lifestyle Wellness Strategic Plan*. Haley provides this information to her virtual assistant to complete her *LWI Statement Tracking template*.

Sheila takes photos of her meals and snacks each day and evaluates how well she has aligned with her 60 percent nutrition *Interim Goal* each week. She uses a whole food, plant-based meal service to make achieving 60 percent easy. She also uses a food journal to record her daily evaluation, reflect, and identify successes and opportunities. This helps with completing her *LWI Statement Tracking template* weekly.

To monitor my sleep quality, I make a mental note of my sleep quality milestone times:1) my wake-sleep time when I turn out the lights, 2) if I had an extended wake-sleep duration, my sleep-period time(s) I wake during the night, 4) my sleep-wake time when I get out of bed. While waiting for my tea to brew, I rate my sleep quality and how I am feeling. I also note if I had any quality deviations and extended gaps between sleep periods and note the adjustments I will make. I've been at this for some time now, so I compile my *LWI Statement Tracking template* quarterly but still note my sleep quality measures weekly.

✦ ✦ ✦

Your goal is to find what works for you and what you can consistently commit to using. My first measurement plan did not work out well. It was still focused daily on individual tasks versus mindset, quality, and return on my wellness investment. I purchased a large calendar whiteboard and used a different color marker for each lifestyle wellness component. When I felt I achieved my daily goal for each component, I added a colored star on that day. At the end of the month, I documented the percentage of days I had achieved my goal for each component, identified areas of concern, and adjusted my tactics. That sounds great, right? Not necessarily. Instead of focusing on forward progress, I was focused more on the past, what I had done or not done. I was not embracing my imperfect self, living my beliefs about achieving my fantastic wellness future: my be, do, have. Instead, I was embracing my perfectionist self: my wasn't, didn't do, failed, which opened the door for my negative feelings to drive my future behaviors. This doesn't work in the long term.

My thoughts went negative, focusing on the gaps and the days I failed to meet my goals. I would beat myself up so I would do better the next day, which did not typically work, instead of staying neutral and choosing to celebrate mindset growth, awareness, and experimentation. When you think negative thoughts, the brain makes it more difficult to change. Confidence is a skill that is learned and practiced. When you think confident thoughts, you behave in a confident manner—you make stuff happen—thinking and belief beget action. The mind tells the body what to do. I have since transitioned to a journal and document perceived quality for the *Future Targets* aligned with the *EBQSs* for each component. Lifestyle wellness is the way I live life every day. At the end of this year, I plan to change my LWI evaluation frequency to every six months. This is because I've already achieved many of my *Future Targets* and am on autopilot, so less frequent evaluation is required (notice I wrote less frequent, not no evaluation).

Creating an effective measurement and evaluation process that focuses on growth, evolving mindset, and tangible internal benefits that lower long-term disease progression risk versus focusing on gaps and deficiencies is a critical component of your *Lifestyle Wellness Strategic Plan*. It should not be glossed over quickly. Without an effective measurement process, you may end up spinning your wheels or taking the wrong path and not realize it until you've given up or reverted to past unhealthy habits. Your measurement and evaluation process helps you read the road signs along your journey, take a detour when needed, and change routes completely when necessary; you always know if you are heading in the right direction toward your *Wellness Vision* and optimizing your wellness investment. It's up to you to determine how you will measure your progress toward your goals and targets. Use what works for you and know that, when your healthy behaviors become your default, standard operating procedures in your life, less frequent measurement may be required. You just know, and you just do! What you measure matters. If you don't measure it, it doesn't matter. Achieving your desired health and wellness *does* matter. Treat it as if it is as important as, or even more important than, your wealth. I suggest not waiting to experience having one and not the other.

Dr. Lori's Insights

- Don't end up with a hefty financial portfolio but an empty lifestyle wellness portfolio; reap the benefits of your investment in your health and wellness now without any early withdrawal penalties and taxes.
- Stay focused on evolving your Well-Leader Mindset™. A Well-Leader focuses on future possibilities and knows how to use the conscious mind to overpower the nay-saying subconscious thoughts that get in the way.
- The best tracking system is the one you actually use! Find what works easily for you. If you are a paper person, stick with journaling and tracking on paper or use tasks on your calendar.
- Don't take your failures with your wellness (or anything) personally; they do not define you or your worth/value. Separate yourself from your failures—use them as growth opportunities to experiment, have fun, and try something new.

CHAPTER EIGHTEEN

Defending Your Future Focus

It is almost guaranteed that life will interrupt your health and wellness journey, no matter what you try to do—that's simply part of being human. How will you be ready to defend yourself against life situations that test your thoughts and beliefs and be ready to manage conditions that attempt to disrupt your future focus, motivation, and resilience? Continuing to evolve your Well-Leader Mindset™ and cultivating resilience to weather life's storms will keep you moving forward. It's about maintaining a growth mindset that focuses on possibilities by actively choosing how to think about a situation and using every opportunity as a learning moment. You reframe your story to what you want it to be. It's about not focusing on the past or feeling that you are a victim of your environment; you can't change the past, and being a victim puts you in a powerless place. It's about staying mindful and aware of your thinking and recognizing when to adapt and change (and not give up) in the face of challenges or when things don't seem to be working. Things may not be working out for a reason; find the reason, change your thinking, and move past it or move forward with it.

Until I started my lifestyle wellness journey, I had been living in my past and always felt like a victim of my circumstances. Why were these things happening to me? What did I do to deserve this? I spent most of my time and energy trying to fix and control all the external things in order to feel happier, more confident, and more successful at work and with my own health and wellness. The more I stayed in victim mode, the more things I found in my life to validate my feelings of oppression and victimhood. I often felt frustrated, as though I was broken in some way. I had accepted that struggling with my health and wellness was as good as it would get for me, something that I would have to deal with and accept for the rest of my life. Being the introvert I am, I hid my feelings from everyone and did the best I could to stay motivated, positive, and forward-focused.

Then, in November of 2016, my father suffered his heart attack. I initially viewed this as a sad, negative event; however, I realize now that this event ignited my *calling*. Downsizing and moving back to Pennsylvania to nurture and support my parents gave me the opportunity to step back and figure myself out concurrently. This took my focus off the negativity of the past and shifted my perspective; what did I want this situation to mean? Through my certification journey, finding lifestyle medicine, and embarking on my own journey toward achieving my *Wellness Vision*, I realized that my power came from within—by managing my thoughts and beliefs about what I choose for my future. By doing so, I create the experiences I desire and generate a ripple effect. I improve the life and health of those around me, they affect the health and wellness of others, and so on. I've learned not to get caught up in what other people think or say; I can't control what they think, and that's okay. I only control my own thoughts, beliefs, and actions. I choose to stand tall and confident in my *Wellness Nonconformist* skin. The health and wellness changes you've decided to make and the resilience required to sustain your changes start in your brain. You decide, believe it, and then own it. You will have normal ups and downs to keep life interesting—the contrast helps us appreciate the positive experiences much more. The key is you choosing what you want those ups and downs to mean to you and then living it!

In the past, when you felt you got off track with your wellness or *fell off the wagon*, how did you respond? Did you:

- Beat yourself up, dwell on your perceived self-failure, and let your negative thoughts drain your energy and motivation even more, enough to quit?
  Or
- Stay aware and in the moment, acknowledge your feelings and be okay with them, reflect upon what happened, and reframe and regain control to move forward and get back on track?

It's normal for everyone to have a slip or skip. You may have an *oops* moment or rationalize an unhealthy choice at times. That's okay; it's more important how you think about it and what you do next. Your brain is wired to focus on the negative. It's called *negativity bias*; it's just what your brain does if you let it. As a result, you are over-focused on the negative, which does not help defend your future focus. Your *LWI* tracking process provides a visual indication when slips and negative feelings linger too long and put you at risk for a lapse in which old thinking and behaviors begin to emerge. Lapses may lead to relapses unless you recognize and manage your thinking early on. Lapses are short, but relapses last longer, during which unhealthy thinking and behaviors may take hold again. Feelings follow focus, and focus follows feelings. If you focus on the negativity of your slip, skip, or lapse and think you are a failure, you are, and you may progress to feeling defeated, stuck, or not strong enough. If you use the opportunity as a learning moment by staying aware and changing your thoughts about the situation to put you back in control, your focus will be on adapting, brainstorming replacement behaviors, and staying energized so you can continue to move forward.

That's why it is vital to include resilience tactics in your *Lifestyle Wellness Strategic Plan*, to prop you up when your old automatic thoughts and feelings attempt to hijack your progress when normal skips and slips happen. You get to design your resilience tactics to help you stop the thoughts that lead to negative feelings in their tracks (snap), work through the negativity, and then construct new helpful meanings, which change your perspective and beliefs about your wellness future. The past is not your future story; if you stay in the past, you will become nothing more. Your resilience tactics, represented by the following equation, ensure you stay attentive to your current thinking and beliefs and efficiently interpret and reframe your experience. This gives you back your power by turning the experience into a possibility-focused, positive learning opportunity.

$$\text{Attention} + \text{Thinking \& Beliefs} = \text{Experience}$$

Staying focused on your thinking, not your feelings or the situation, helps you become more resilient overall. Different events may cause the same feelings. Having a strategy to recognize your negativity bias, change your thinking, and maintain resilience during these times can be used regardless of the situation. Viewing life challenges as opportunities to call upon your resilience tactics that align with your strengths allows you to flex your creativity and problem-solving abilities to move forward with healthy lifestyle decisions that support your *Wellness Vision*. You've gotten to where you are now as a successful leader by facing challenges head on. It's no different with your health and wellness.

Throughout this planning process, you've learned about yourself and applied the strategic wellness activities to create a solid foundation to build upon, sustain, and defend your wellness future. First, your *Wellness Why*, *Wellness Authenticity*, and *Wellness Presence* support your foundation. Next, the positive transition process, the behavior mourning process, and the planning process to balance your tactics to focus on your *Wellness Vision* support your resilience. Finally, exercising your growth, investor mindset changes how you interpret what you experience when facing challenges. You've committed to investing in the long-term wealth of your health by giving yourself the gift of wellness in the present and beyond. So, to keep you moving toward and defending your wellness future, you get to create your resilience tactics. These tactics increase awareness and combat faulty thinking before it happens to keep your health and wellness investing efforts on track. This focuses your attention on the thoughts and beliefs that reduce the negativity bias and instead feed your positive energy and motivation. You experience life challenges in a whole new way and may even look forward to them so you can flex your creativity ... bring it!

Strategic Wellness Activities

The strategic wellness activities in this chapter guide you through identifying the thoughts, beliefs, and feelings that may put you at risk for negativity bias that could lead to lapses and relapses along your lifelong strategic wellness journey. You won't identify situations or events but focus on the feelings and emotions that arise when you let your guard down and allow external events, challenges, and circumstances to take over and guide your life. You identify the resilience tactics and support that will keep you on track with your wellness journey when life tries to get in your way.

1. **Complete Section 7.0 My Lifestyle Wellness Resilience Tactics section in your** *Lifestyle Wellness Strategic Plan.*
    Review the items in the Resilience Checklist and create a Mindset & Thinking Change Tactic for each. Follow the instructions in the investment guide to complete the checklist.
2. **Keep your resilience tactics handy for when you need them.**
    And you will need them. It takes time and practice to implant new mindset and resilience tactics. Until then, write your tactics on a card you keep in your pocket or a note in your phone.
3. **Complete the Courage & Confidence Check.**
    How do you want to feel living your best life? Did you create effective resilience tactics to stop your brain in its tracks when it starts to go negative? Do your resilience tactics represent the version of you who has become courageous and confident in defending and investing in your long-term wellness future?

WLM in Practice

Haley relied on her spouse to help keep her moving forward when she felt stressed and needed support. They planned time each day to sit together, talk about current work issues, and create a plan for moving forward. Her husband kept her on track with her nutrition by preparing healthful meals to prevent her from slipping back to eating junk food and prepackaged, processed foods.

Sheila committed to using her *Wellness Presence* activity when she started focusing too much on the negativity of the past and arguing for her limitations. She developed five key beliefs she would repeat as her mirror conversation when the thoughts crept back into her consciousness. She linked a short activity to each belief and repeated the activity throughout the day until she was able to move forward. She had an accountability buddy in her workplace to call on for support and encouragement as well.

When Marjorie felt her enthusiasm about her self-care wane during the day, she took a five to ten minute walking meditation break to calm her thinking. During her walk, she visualized her future self in her mind and recited her *Wellness Vision*. Practicing seeing herself in the future gets her through the rough patch and reignites her energy and enthusiasm to defend and invest in her health and wellness future.

✦ ✦ ✦

I've had to call upon my resilience tactics often along my health and wellness journey, and I imagine I will continue to do so. A tactic I implement daily to counter my normal fluctuation in enthusiasm, energy, and focus in the late morning and mid-afternoon is engaging in one of my five-minute *Expresso yoga* routines using my subscription yoga app. There are over fifty routines to choose from, depending on how I feel and what I want to focus on. My favorites are *Endorphin Booster* and *Flow & Activate*. You most likely experience similar peaks and troughs in energy and focus throughout the day. These are called ultradian rhythms and are completely normal. The premise is that our bodies go through alternating periods of rest and activity and that each full rest-activity cycle lasts between 80–120 minutes. During the day, this feels like low energy, loss of focus or motivation, and exhaustion.[115] Instead of medicating the normal troughs in my ultradian rhythm with caffeine or sugar, I choose movement and stretching for five-to-ten minutes. Works every time.

Having resilience tactics to use in all areas of your life gives you the courage and confidence to manage what life throws your way. It truly is all about how you think and manage your thoughts. You've most likely heard the quote by the poet John Milton, "The mind is its own place and in itself, can make a Heaven of Hell, or a Hell of Heaven." I decided I wanted to finally be well and be a wellness role model, even though I was far from it. The more I thought about it, the more I felt it. The more I felt it, the more I believed it and engaged in actions that would create it. The more I engaged in actions to create it, the more I achieved it. You get the picture. Don't let your current thinking hold you back. There is no set time for making a change; let it take as long as it needs for you to buy in, believe you can achieve it, and then act. Your ability to achieve your authentic wellness exists right now, so step in, claim it, and then fiercely defend it.

---

[115] Buzzard, "*Avoid Burnout and Increase Awareness Using Ultradian Rhythms.*"

Dr. Lori's Insights

- Resilience tactics help us get out of our default mode of thinking. You decide how you want to think. Re-focus your brain on pleasure, novelty, and enjoyment to quickly move past the negativity bias, regret, and self-criticism.
- Where attention goes, energy flows. Focus your attention on resilience, which creates emotional agility: the ability to demonstrate flexibility in dealing with emotions and life challenges.
- All your power is about constructing your thoughts around what you want to think about your past and, more importantly, your future. Then live it.

CHAPTER NINETEEN

Your Gift to Keep on Giving & Getting

Congratulations, you're in the home stretch of completing your *Lifestyle Wellness Strategic Plan*. When you begin implementing your plan, every day is a new day to move forward and transform your Well-Leader Mindset™. Your lifestyle wellness is an investment in your future and a work in progress for the rest of your life. As you live your best self, you will continue to monitor, adjust, and enhance your plan to keep it relevant to your stage of life and advance your mindset.

This is how you continue to *give* yourself—and keep *getting*—the gift of wellness.

Lifestyle wellness is a lifelong journey. Relax, settle in, and enjoy the journey—the ups and downs and all. It is the gift you keep getting every time you implement the tactics and distractions in your plan and make healthy lifestyle choices your default. The key is to set up your healthy lifestyle in a way that works for your life and keep experimenting, which is what you've done throughout the process of creating your *Lifestyle Wellness Strategic Plan*. You learned that becoming a *Wellness Nonconformist* can be challenging; you may experience uncomfortable thoughts and feelings when implementing your healthy actions, especially around unhealthy people. These feelings mean you are on the right track; you are on your way to extraordinary, not ordinary! Your Well-Leader Mindset™ is evolving.

Working with my clients, I've found several factors that predict success in making sustained changes related to thinking, beliefs, and behavior that support health and wellness:

- You have a clear, personal *Wellness Why* that justifies your strong desire to make changes.
- You believe you have the necessary skills, courage, confidence, and support to make the changes.
- Your *Wellness Vision* of your best self and what you see yourself doing in the future are aligned with your strengths and evidence-based standards.
- You are open to possibilities related to your health goals and believe the changes will be beneficial and contribute to you achieving your best self.
- You have minimized obstacles in your thinking and your physical and social environments to make the changes you desire.
- You have a written plan that contains measurement strategies and tactics to strengthen your resilience. (Note: documenting your plan increases your success rate to 80 percent.)
- You have the support and encouragement from people you value and the community support and resources you desire (Note: making your plan social can increase your success rate to 100 percent.)

You have achieved all these steps except for the last one—gathering the ongoing support, encouragement, community, and resources to seamlessly implement your plan. It's time to put the finishing touches on your *Lifestyle Wellness Strategic Plan* so you can, and you will move forward on your lifetime wellness journey courageously and confidently and begin optimizing the return on your wellness investment now and in retirement!

The strategic wellness activities in this chapter help you finalize your *Lifestyle Wellness Strategic Plan* by creating your sustainment tactics, which include determining next steps on how to proceed and securing external resources and support to keep you courageously and confidently moving forward. You may decide you want to work with me as your *Leadership Wellness Strategist* to continue your momentum and enroll in one of my Well-Leader Mindset™ Strategic Progression support programs to continue your mindset progression and support the implementation of your *Lifestyle Wellness Strategic Plan* to sustain your wellness journey into the future. My programs provide support from certified professionals including board-certified health and wellness coaches, nutritional consultants, fitness trainers, herbalists, holistic practitioners, mindset coaches, etc., based on your specific wellness support and sustainment requirements.

You may choose to set up a whole food, plant-based meal delivery service, purchase equipment or technology, rearrange your home and office furniture, join a gym and engage with a support community. This is the time to get your support systems and resources set up *before* you get started and find yourself struggling and feeling overwhelmed. You know you, and you know the *must haves* that need to be in place for you to be successful. This is important stuff! We are talking about elevating your health to the same level as your wealth; it's not the time to skimp, nickel-and-dime things, and cut corners. *Invest* in yourself, optimize your *Lifestyle Wellness Index (LWI)*, and set yourself up to be successful. What is the incredible health and wellness you get to achieve worth to you?

Strategic Wellness Activities

The strategic wellness activities in this chapter put the finishing touches on your plan, so you get to solidify your belief that your *Wellness Vision* is possible now and feel courageous and confident you have a solid path forward.

1. **Complete Section 8.0 My Lifestyle Wellness Sustainment Tactics in your *Lifestyle Wellness Strategic Plan.***
   Identify and document next steps and resources to initiate before you implement your plan or to engage within the first month. Review the sustainment resource guide on the book resource website for suggestions.

2. **Complete Section 9.0 My Lifestyle Wellness Strategy Planning Insights & Guiding Practices in your *Lifestyle Wellness Strategic Plan.***
   Reflect on how your energy, focus, and perceptions have changed as you've moved through this wellness strategic planning process. Record key insights that will guide your thinking, beliefs, and actions going forward.

3. **Complete Section 10.0 My Lifestyle Wellness Strategy Session Insights in your *Lifestyle Wellness Strategic Plan.***
   Use this section to record additional insights and key takeaways from wellness strategy sessions and from collaboration with your Well-Leader peers in my social media groups and programs. Ongoing engagement will support your forward progress and ensure your plan remains *alive* and *breathing*!

4. **Confirm your plan implementation start date.**
   Choose an official start date to *fully* implement your plan. You may have already started implementing some of your tactics and distractions. It's time to get *officially* started when you have your initial external support resources in place.

5. **Complete the Final Courage & Confidence Check.**
   How ready are you to step into your authentic wellness and begin living your best life by optimizing your investment in your long-term health and wellness? Are you ready to accept your lifelong challenge to increase your lifespan and your health span? Did you do the work to feel confident that your completed *Lifestyle Wellness Strategic Plan* represents *you*—the version of you who feels authentic, courageous, and confident in your ability to invest in your long-term

wellness future? This version of you isn't in the distance. She/he is right in front of you; step into your authentic wellness!

WLM in Practice

You decide on your next steps and when you are ready to implement your plan. Do you still have groundwork you are planning to finish, or is 80 percent in place to implement now? Don't wait too long to get started; 80 percent is good enough because plans constantly evolve and change. Haley got started immediately. She purchased a treadmill, redesigned her home environment to encourage movement throughout the day, initiated a whole food, plant-based meal delivery service, and purchased a standing desk and a light therapy lamp for her office. She focused on reorganizing her workdays and used her virtual assistant to schedule all her health and wellness appointments.

Sheila joined a yoga studio, initiated a whole food, plant-based meal delivery service at work, and moved her elliptical machine to her den. She uses it for reading and watching videos in the evening. She redesigned her sleeping area to include room darkening shades, red night lights, and a white noise maker. She established a power-down hour before bed to relax, have a cup of tea, and calm her mind before sleep.

Marjorie wanted to learn more about the healing powers of herbal medicine. I connected her with an herbalist in my resource network, who provides collaboration and resources via social media and virtual support programs to address Marjorie's specific conditions and concerns.

◆ ◆ ◆

When I implemented my strategy five years ago, I felt that I was only about 50–75 percent there. I would have to figure out the rest along the way as I experimented with what worked and did not work. I didn't want to stay stuck in analysis paralysis or get caught up in my cycle of perfection. Even now, as the fund manager of my *LWI*, I adapt and make changes to my tactics and distractions, sometimes daily, to continue to optimize my long-term wellness investments. So don't keep spinning or stagnating; it's okay to allow your stocks (tactics and distractions) to fluctuate daily until you find the combination that feels authentic. Remember, the *Evidence-Based Quality Standards* for the lifestyle wellness components may not change, but your tactics and distractions *will* change as your mindset evolves and as circumstances change. I'm hopeful you will use the book resource website and support in my social media group to continue to elevate your Well-Leader Mindset™ and inspire you to take more action. You never outperform your beliefs, so continue to raise your wellness possibilities ceiling using deliberate small steps, tactics, and distractions in your plan that align with your strengths and keep your journey feeling authentic.

At this point, it may be helpful for you to step back from your planning and reflect on your work. This helps you relax your mind and refocus. Then revisit your *Lifestyle Wellness Strategic Plan* to review it end-to-end and make final changes, identify additional next steps, and gather more support to implement your plan. You may realize that ongoing support is the key to helping you feel confident your plan is ready. Ongoing participation with other Well-Leaders in our programs and social media group can enhance your courage and motivation as well. Periodic wellness strategy sessions and weekly program support are also effective ways to enhance the implementation of your plan as you embark on your journey toward your *Wellness Vision*.

Making and sustaining changes often feels exhausting. Along your lifelong wellness journey, plan for periodic stops at rest areas to enjoy time to relax and regenerate. As I mentioned earlier, ongoing strategy sessions and weekly group support activities offer a safe place to sort through your challenges, refocus your mindset, and explore your progress. Engaging with like-minded, Well-Leaders on the same journey as you facilitates sharing better routes around detours, challenges, and roadblocks along the way. Start your investment in your wellness future off right by getting the support you desire and staying connected; no cutting corners this time!

Dr. Lori's Insights

- When you implement your plan, you focus on experiments vs. perfection. Take a chance and implement when you feel your plan is at 80 percent. Not everything is going to work as is. Keep experimenting until you find what works for you.
- Decisions move your life forward; decide ahead of time that you get to be fine, no matter what you choose. Then, seek the evidence to support your new way of being. Your identity must support your new *being-ness*!
- The sooner you implement, the sooner you begin replacing old, recycled, looping thoughts that have not been serving you with new beliefs, thinking, and actions that reflect the Well Leader you are—right now!

CHAPTER TWENTY

Well-Leader Mindset™–Your New Beginning

Woo-hoo! It's great to see you here! I knew I would. You must feel excited and energized right now—you have a solid strategic plan to finally achieve and sustain the wellness you desire and start living your best life. When you implement your *Lifestyle Wellness Strategic Plan*, keep it accessible and use your *WLM Investment Guide* and additional tools, templates, and guidance provided on the book resource website to keep you on track. You will have access to the website for life, as well as access to my Well-Leader Mindset™ LinkedIn group. At first, it may help to post your tactics and distractions where you can see them every day, schedule them on your calendar, and use reminders. Your plan will soon become encoded in your mind and your life.

Transforming to a Well-Leader Mindset™ involves having attitudes, beliefs, and expectations about your health and wellness that create the foundation of who you are and how you think. This influences how you lead and prioritize your self-care, inspire others to improve their health and well-being, and act as a wellness role model when you interact and engage with others in your network. This mindset is important to hone because it impacts all components of your work and home life. As your Well-Leader Mindset™ progresses and your beliefs about your ability to achieve the health and wellness you desire change, the tactics and distractions in your plan will become a part of your new way to think, behave, and live. Remember, lifestyle wellness is a journey, not a destination; you are investing in long-term wellness for you (and those with whom you engage) to enjoy in the present, in retirement, and beyond. As your life situation changes and you encounter turns and bumps along the road, you call upon your resilience tactics and support systems to adapt your plan to defend and maintain your forward focus toward your *Wellness Vision*.

I want to recognize the incredible commitment and effort you've put forth creating your *Lifestyle Wellness Strategic Plan*. It takes someone like you with strong beliefs and convictions to stick with it; your long-term health and wellness is important to you. You are starting out where *you* are, and this is all right. *You are at the beginning of your new beginning!* You have your whole life to practice (and sometimes fail), learn, and adapt; consistently practicing what makes your journey authentic makes it permanent until it's time to adapt again and yet again. You will feel more courageous, confident, and capable every day and will soon experience what optimizing the return on your wellness investment feels like; the value of your *Lifestyle Wellness Index* will skyrocket! It's time to believe you *do* have the knowledge, skills, courage, and confidence to move forward on your wellness journey of a lifetime! However, please know that I will be here for you now and in the future. Please visit my website at www.loriuslifestyle.com to learn more about how I can support you and how to keep your momentum going by enrolling in one of my Well-Leader Mindset™ Strategic Progression support programs. Feel free to join my Well-Leader Mindset™ LinkedIn group to post strategic wellness questions, view weekly information, updated research, and program offers, and enjoy opportunities to engage with other Well-Leaders like yourself.

I thought long and hard about how to bring your amazing strategic planning work to a close and propel you forward on the transformational lifestyle wellness journey that awaits you. A checklist about next steps seemed too simplistic—you already know the next steps that will work for you. I then considered an oath, but again, it seemed too simplistic; an oath is really just an affirmed statement or promise. Neither felt like *enough*, nor did they speak to the evolving Well-Leader Mindset™ that I know is critical to inspire you to invest for a lifetime in the long-term health and wellness you envision. I began searching for a closing that would convey the importance of how changing your mindset and establishing your new thinking and belief patterns about your health and wellness will be the only way to get you unstuck and give you the ongoing courage and confidence to change your life. That's it, a creed—a *Well-Leader Mindset™ Creed*!

The definitions of *creed* that seem to fit what I wanted to convey are: 1) any system, doctrine, or codification of beliefs;[116] 2) a philosophy or a particular belief system that guides behaviors.[117] The *Well-Leader Mindset™ Creed* presents ten self-beliefs that foster the thinking to elevate your commitment to enhancing and defending your strategic *Wellness Vision*. Your beliefs (good, bad, or neutral) create your thoughts, which elicit emotions and feelings which guide your actions and inactions.

---

[116] Dictionary.com, "*Creed*."
[117] Vocabulary.com, "*Creed*."

When you start with creating new guiding beliefs, your thinking, feelings, and permanent change follow. Through your thoughtful work, you have begun changing your beliefs and have integrated them throughout your *Lifestyle Wellness Strategic Plan*. When you implement your plan, you get to live your new beliefs and act courageously and confidently in your pursuit of extraordinary health and wellness. Are you ready to accept, affirm, and verbalize your guiding beliefs using the *Well-Leader Mindset™ Creed*?

Well-Leader Mindset™ Creed

Please recite with me:

- I believe I have the ability to give myself the gift of health and wellness and that my self-care is a top priority in my life.
- I believe I am not at the mercy of my genetics; I can and I will control my health and wellness destiny.
- I believe I have uncovered my true *Wellness Why*, the *Why* that controls my thinking, elicits strong positive emotions, and drives my new thoughts and behaviors.
- I believe I already possess the strengths and values to live my best self; I am confident I know how to use them to strengthen my *Wellness Presence* and make my wellness journey feel authentic, enthusiastic, and engaging.
- I believe I have everything to gain from achieving the long-term health and wellness I desire; I understand the importance of transitioning my beliefs and thinking first before attempting to change my behaviors.
- I believe I have a clear, unencumbered *Wellness Vision* that provides a compelling description of me at my best self; I actively think about my vision every day to change my thinking and change my life; I view failure as an opportunity to learn, expand my possibilities, and achieve even more.
- I believe I have aligned my lifestyle wellness strategy with my *Wellness Vision*. I believe my tactics and distractions are enough to achieve my *Future Targets*; I can and I will do the work to make my vision a reality.
- I believe my health is as important as my wealth, and I treat my strategic lifestyle wellness as a long-term investment in myself and my legacy. I focus on optimizing my return on my health and wellness investments and monitor and manage my investment wisely.
- I believe I can manage my external circumstances. I have the power inside of me to manage my thoughts and create the experiences I desire. I believe the health and wellness changes I

experience create a ripple effect and impact others in positive ways.

- I believe it is my duty to live my best life and empower others to better well-being. I believe I am an effective health and wellness role model who advocates for lifestyle wellness at home and in my organization.

Strategic Wellness Activities

Do you feel the power of your new thinking? Don't squander the *power* you are feeling right now—get started on your wellness journey today. Don't find yourself a year from now wishing you would have started today! Commit the *Well-Leader Mindset™ Creed* to memory. I've included a printable version of the creed on the book resource website for you to download, frame, and hang on your wall. There is a smaller version for you to print, laminate, and carry with you or snap a photo to use when you need a wellness mindset boost.

1. **Reflect on your Well-Leader Mindset™ transformation.**
   In your investment guide, review each belief in the creed and rate the alignment of your current thinking. For areas rated lower than 80 percent alignment, review the associated chapter(s) and activities or schedule a strategy session to achieve clarity and alignment. What can you do to increase your beliefs alignment?

2. **Finalize your plan and step into your authentic wellness!**
   You can, you will, and you get to be the Well-Leader you envision. When you witness yourself stepping forward into your *Wellness Vision*, you not only see yourself differently, but you also change your life. When you control your thinking and actions, you give yourself the personal power to achieve your vision, despite what is going on in the external world. Your successful transformation to a Well-Leader Mindset™ occurs first at the thought and feeling level of your brain and then authentic actions follow.

3. **Recite the *Well-Leader Mindset™ Creed* daily and whenever you feel your courage and confidence wane.**
   The creed continues to solidify your new beliefs and thinking in your subconscious and crowd out old, limiting thoughts. Keeping the creed in view reminds you that your new beliefs and thinking are driving your behaviors—not the media, other people, or external events. You can't control these; you can only control how you think about them. This keeps your emotions in check and allows you to take action that supports your health and wellness every day. Your beliefs and thinking help you "Be It" first in your mind, then "Do It," and then "Have It," so you experience the outcomes you desire.

Go Forth. Your Possibilities Await!

Five years ago, when my wellness hit rock-bottom and I experienced my wake-up call, I never could have imagined I would be where I am now—reaching an incredible level of health and wellness that *feels authentic to me* and writing this book for you to do the same. As my father would say when he was thanked for his WWII military service, "It was an honor." I echo his statement. It has been an honor to serve you and share my story with you. My belief is that this book and my story inspire you to take immediate action toward achieving the health and wellness you desire and have the ability to achieve *today*! Your people need you, they need your health and wellness legacy. They want you to be around for a long while—engaged, energetic and in great health. That's what I discovered. As my *Lifestyle Wellness Index* increased, the more authentic my beliefs about my health and wellness became. As I achieved a higher level of wellness, I advanced my Well-Leader Mindset™. As my mindset advanced, the better I was at taking care of myself and advocating for my people. By my actions and engagement, I became an inspiring role model for others. Your health and wellness can become an unstoppable chain of events that keeps snowballing!

I can't say it has been easy street and all fun and games. It never will be; I'm sure life has more in store for me, good and bad. The difference now is my Well-Leader Mindset™ has shifted. I have my beliefs and my plan to guide me, and I embrace and am open to *new possibilities* and *nonconformity*. Interestingly, I learned from my mindset coach that the subconscious brain automatically interprets new and different as danger and, if unmanaged, quickly elicits associated emotions and feelings unless you deliberately tell it not to. If you let your subconscious stay in control and do not actively transform your Well-Leader Mindset™, negativity bias will kick back in and you will spiral back into old habits and sad places. I experienced that when my father passed away. I knew my grief and sadness were normal.

I had studied the stages of grieving in nursing school yet found myself stuck somewhere between anger, bargaining, and depression. I had let my emotions and negativity bias overtake me by focusing on regrets—the things I should have said and done—becoming angry over how I had failed and wishing I'd had more time to do things differently. My mindset coach taught me that regret is a *fierce* emotion. It's not helpful most of the time, and it feels heavy and constricting and sabotages growth.

It wasn't until I decided to invest in myself and take a risk that my subconscious brain automatically interpreted my action as *danger*. However, that risk helped me find *my people*—the ones who inspired me to write this book and share my story, the people who inspire me daily to show up differently, think differently, and reconstruct my beliefs to change my thinking and my future. I learned that you don't get over your past, you become who you are *because* of your past. This rings true for me. What did I want my past to mean? I am here because of all the positive and negative experiences I've had, all the people I've influenced and supported, and all those who have supported and inspired me.

I have a very different future to write—a new story to tell and more people to inspire and support, including you!

Think about your own past. What do you want it to mean for you? How can you use it to inspire yourself toward new wellness possibilities? You have your *Lifestyle Wellness Strategic Plan*, you've begun your Well-Leader Mindset™ transformation, and you know I am here to support you. All that's left for you is to step into your authentic future self who is already standing right in front of you. This feels like a great time for a parting *future pull* to keep you believing forward. As you recall from Chapter 5, a future pull is a visualization activity in which you talk about yourself in the future as if it were the present. I describe my future pull in the following epilogue, and guess what, *you are in it*. You are standing in front of me in the future. I will see you soon. Godspeed!

Dr. Lori's Insights

- It's all about *your* mindset. Nothing outside of you has to change for you to achieve the health and wellness you desire. When you stop trying to fix your external environment and other people, and instead, manage your own mind to shift your perception, you experience a life of endless possibilities.
- Keep your *Wellness Vision* in clear sight. It creates the positivity and energy to keep you moving forward in your wellness journey. Unhealthy thoughts that drive unhealthy emotions and create unhealthy habits are a thing of the past!
- Enjoy the feeling of creating forward movement toward your best self. Bask in the feeling that you have a solid roadmap forward!

Epilogue: Join Me in My Future Pull

I t is January 2027, five years into the future and almost ten years from when I began my career transformation and health and wellness journey. I am hosting my first annual Well-Leader Mindset™ Retreat with a large group of incredible Well-Leaders in attendance. I'm well into my 60s, and I've never felt more fit, energetic, and healthy. I completed my welcome address, including the group recitation of the *Well-Leader Mindset™ Creed*. The applause feels amazing yet a bit overwhelming and humbling; it's hard to believe that my strategic wellness investment movement has touched so many amazing, caring, forward-thinking leaders.

I see numerous clients in the audience. They look great—fit, healthy, confident, courageous, and energetic. They accepted the challenge to create the strategic lifestyle of wellness that felt authentic to them. Their *Lifestyle Wellness Index* retirement strategies are solid. They have become the wellness role models and advocates they envisioned. I've supported hundreds of leaders on the same journey, many who have gone on to implement lifestyle medicine practices in their organizations to pay it forward—the ripple effect created by acting on their duty to enhance the health and well-being of their employees. Their organizations have achieved the *Well-Leader Mindset™ Culture Certification*. Wellness has become an integral part of their organization's leadership development curriculum.

Lifestyle wellness noticeably permeates throughout the organization's top-down culture of well-being. They report higher productivity, less absenteeism, and greater employee engagement and retention. Their health insurance claims have decreased, employees are engaging with health plan preventative and wellness services and programs, and they report better physical and emotional health.

Through my Well-Leader Mindset™ movement and the unwavering efforts of the American College of Lifestyle Medicine, key lifestyle medicine legends, lifestyle medicine diplomates, advocates, and practitioners, we have increased the percentage of people in the United States engaging in all four healthy behaviors well *above* the 3% mark. This increase has considerably decreased deaths from chronic diseases of lifestyle and has reduced many of the negative environmental impacts related to our dietary practices. Countless practitioners and hospitals around the world now align their patient care practices and programs with lifestyle medicine, especially whole food, plant-based nutrition; food is medicine. What incredible achievements; however, there is still a lot of work to be done.

I leave the stage and enter the lobby area to begin my book signing. The line is already quite long—a succession of all those leaders ready to embark on their Well-Leader Mindset™ transformation. I think back to my life-changing day in January 2018 sitting in a similar lobby. I quietly and thoughtfully observe retreat participants walking by; they look healthy, fit, and energetic, engaged in lively conversation. I could never have imagined I would be here today. I changed my destiny and ended my wellness cognitive dissonance by investing in my health and wellness and making it a strategic, long-term priority using lifestyle medicine practices. My husband, who is assisting with my book signing, is waiting at the table. He and my dog, Luna, willingly signed up and embarked on the journey with me. Their never-ending support and energy kept me going and expanded my thinking and the endless possibilities I see.

I think about my father's last four years of life and how he willingly accepted my support and embraced lifestyle medicine practices. He never gave up. He inspired me not to give up my quest for the health and wellness I desire and to accept with honor this opportunity to lead and inspire others. All I can think now is, *I'm not done yet!* While basking in this incredible moment, I see *you* walking toward me. You look amazing! I see wellness, courage, and confidence radiating from you as you approach. I see that you, too, chose the fork in the road to change your health and wellness destiny; you've continued your journey to become a Well-Leader and your best self. We greet each other warmly and, after a few minutes of conversation, I ask you, "When you think about living life at its best, what does it look like for you now?"

You smile and think back to when you were first asked this question—while working on creating your *Wellness Vision* for your *Lifestyle Wellness Strategic Plan*. You immediately implemented your plan, engaging in ongoing support to achieve success. You've since reviewed and updated your plan to accommodate a few key life changes. Your *Lifestyle Wellness Index* is still on track to achieve your *Future Targets* well before retirement. Your people are enjoying your health and wellness legacy now. You take a few moments to think about the question and compile your response. Then you reply, "_____." Press pause....

Before you reply, imagine yourself standing there right now, five years into the future, after having implemented your *Lifestyle Wellness Strategic Plan* and stepping into your authentic wellness. What are you thinking? How do you look and feel? And most importantly, what do you hear yourself saying? Did you accept the challenge unconditionally to change your health and wellness destiny?

Are you living disease free and medication free, focusing on your *Wellness Vision*? Have you become a savvy wellness investor treating your health as important as your wealth by integrating wellness into all areas of your life? Have you become the health and wellness change agent and advocate exerting a positive ripple effect on all those you support and influence? When you commit to transforming your Well-Leader Mindset™, you see that all things *are* possible. Your decisions determine your destiny—decide to change, rewrite your own health and wellness story, and then pass that legacy on to your family, friends, colleagues, team members, and community. All while you reap the benefits in the present and long into your future. Press Play.... So now, what is your reply?

Acknowledgments

I always knew I had a book in me. However, it wasn't until I found my *people*, the people who inspire new possibilities, that my dream became my reality. I am incredibly grateful to my extraordinary coach and consultant, Sara Connell, best-selling author and founder of Thought Leader Academy (www.saraconnell.com), who reenergized my passion for authoring my book. I could not have done it without her guidance and support, the support of my book editor and coach Megan Jackson, the energetic weekly engagement with my fellow TLAers, and the personalized attention of my publisher.

I can't forget my mindset coach, Liz Nicklas (www.liznicklas.com), for igniting my final mindset shift that put the icing on the cake. Working with her and the other incredible women in her Mindset Masterclass solidified my belief that all possibilities are mine and that I can and I will use my pain as my purpose to make the world a better place.

And finally, the American College of Lifestyle Medicine (www.lifestylemedicine.org), my beacon and stabilizing force in a dysfunctional and out-of-control healthcare system. Without the membership, education, certification, and networking support of the incredible legends, board members, practitioners, and engaged members of this organization, who knows where my health and wellness and that of my family would be right now.

About the Author

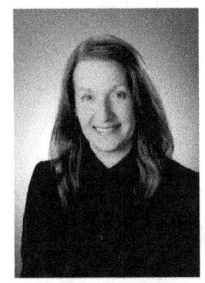

D r. Lori Lindbergh is an I/O psychologist and Wellness Investment Strategist at LORIUS Lifestyle, and creator of the Well-Leader Mindset™ Strategic Progression Framework. Lori was an unwell-leader for over thirty years until she cracked the code to end her *wellness cognitive dissonance* and achieve incredible health and wellness integrating mindset change, business strategy, wellness coaching, and lifestyle medicine aligned with financial investment concepts. Her innovative wellness investing framework helps leaders optimize their health and wellness ROI by stepping into the degree of wellness and chronic disease risk acceptance that feels authentic and fits their lifestyle.

When leaders become well, they understand how to create a ripple effect of well-being in their organizations. Lori's possibilities thinking and her rare combination of education, experience, and board certifications contribute to her unique perspective and thought leadership, which helps her leadership clients get unstuck, quiet their dissonance, and finally become the CEO of their wellness. Lori currently lives in western Pennsylvania with her husband David and their plant-powered dog, Luna. She loves to unleash her creativity in the kitchen by experimenting and preparing whole food, plant-based versions of her favorite meals. Lori is available for keynote speaking, presentations, organizational programs, and strategic wellness workshops. To find out more about Lori, her innovative framework, and how she can support you and your organization visit www.loriuslifestyle.com or www.well-leadermindset.com.

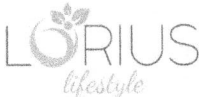

Contact her by email at lori@loriuslifestyle.com or connect via LinkedIn.

Bibliography

Ackerman, Courtney E. "83 Benefits of Journaling for Depression, Anxiety, and Stress." Last modified May 2, 2022. https://positivepsychology.com/benefits-of-journaling/

Alcohol Research Current Reviews Editorial Staff. "Drinking Patterns and Their Definition." Alcohol Research Current Reviews 39, no. 1 (January 2018). https://arcr.niaaa.nih.gov/binge-drinking-predictors-patterns-and-consequences/drinking-patterns-and-their-definitions

American College of Lifestyle Medicine. "Lifestyle Medicine Core Competencies Program." Accessed September-October 2020. https://www.lifestylemedicine.org/ACLM/Education/LMCC/LMCC.aspx?hkey=2d7fc3cd-4b02-45ae-88d3-a88cdeeacb9b

American College of Lifestyle Medicine. "What is Lifestyle Medicine?" Accessed March 5, 2022. https://www.lifestylemedicine.org/ACLM/About/What_is_Lifestyle_Medicine/ACLM/About/What_is_Lifestyle_Medicine_/Lifestyle_Medicine.aspx?hkey=26f3eb6b-8294-4a63-83de-35d429c3bb88

Barnard, Neal. "Why It's So Hard to Give Up Cheese." Last modified May 24, 2017. https://www.forksoverknives.com/wellness/addictive-food-cheese-pizza/

Becker, Karen, and Habib, Rodney. *The Forever Dog: Surprising New Science to Help Your Canine Companion Live Younger, Healthier & Longer.* New York: Harper Wave/Harper Collins, 2021. Kindle.

Bridges, William, and Bridges, Susan. *Managing Transitions: Making the Most of Change.* Lebanon, IN: Da Capo Lifelong Books, 2016. Kindle.

Buzzard, Brad. "Avoid Burnout and Increase Awareness Using Ultradian Rhythms." Last modified November 7, 2017. https://betterhumans.pub/avoid-burnout-and-increase-awareness-using-ultradian-rhythms-5e64158e7e19

Campbell, Thomas. "How Strict Does My Plant-Based Diet Need To Be?" Last modified June 23, 2021. https://nutritionstudies.org/how-strict-does-my-plant-based-diet-need-to-be/?utm_campaign =articles&utm_source=linkedin&utm_medium=social&utm_content= 1624628977

Caprino, Kathy. "The Top 3 Reasons New Year's Resolutions Fail and How Yours Can Succeed." Last modified December 21, 2019. https://www.forbes.com/sites/kathycaprino/2019/12/21/ the-top-3-reasons-new-years-resolutions-fail-and-how-yours-can-succeed/?sh=187a45569929

Centers for Disease Control. "How You Can Prevent Chronic Diseases." Accessed on March 5 2022. https://www.cdc.gov/chronicdisease/about/prevent/index.htm

Compendium of Physical Activities. "Adult Compendium of Physical Activities." Last modified 2011. https://sites.google.com/site/compendiumofphysicalactivities/home?authuser=0

Cuddy, Amy. *Presence: Bringing Your Bolder Self to Your Biggest Challenges*. New York: Little, Brown Spark, 2015. Kindle.

Davison, Courtney. "The No-B.S. Guide to Vegan Protein." Last modified September 26, 2019. https://www.forksoverknives.com/wellness/vegan-protein-guide-athletes/

DeNoon, Daniel J. "7 Rules For Eating." Last modified March 23, 2009 https://www.webmd. com/ food-recipes/news/20090323/7-rules-for-eating

Dictionary.com. Accessed on March 5, 2022. www.dictionary.com

Environmental Working Group. "EWG Verified™." Accessed on March 5, 2022. https://www.ewg. org/ewgverified/

Frates, Beth, Bonnet, Jonathan P., Joseph, Richard, and Peterson, James A. *Lifestyle Medicine Handbook: An Introduction to the Power of Healthy Habits*. Monterey, CA: Healthy Learning, 2019. Kindle.

Fredrickson, Barbara. *Positivity: Discover the Upward Spiral That Will Change Your Life*. New York: Crown Publishing, 2019. Kindle.

Gold, Jamie. *Wellness by Design: A Room-By-Room Guide to Optimizing Your Home For Health, Fitness and Happiness*. New York: Tiller Press, 2021. Kindle.

Greger, Michael. "Shaking the Salt Habit." Last modified April 27, 2016. https://nutritionfacts. org/ video/shaking-salt-habit/

Hallowell, Edward. *Connect: 12 Vital Ties That Open Your Heart, Lengthen Your Life, and Deepen Your Soul*. Toronto: Random House of Canada Limited, 1999. Kindle.

Harvard Health Publishing. "Can Relationships Boost Longevity and Well-Being?" Last modified June 1, 2017. https://www.health.harvar-boost-longevity-and-well-being

Hopper, Elizabeth. "How Your Social Life Might Help You Live Longer." Last modified July 28, 2020. https://greatergood.berkeley.edu/article/item/how_your_social_life_might_help_you_life_longer

Jonas, Steven, and Phillips, Edward. *ACSM's Exercise is Medicine: A clinician's Guide to Exercise Prescription*. Philadelphia, PA: American College of Sports Medicine, 2009. Kindle.

Just Stand.org. "The Facts: The Human Body is Designed to Move." Accessed on March 5, 2022. https://www.juststand.org/the-facts/

Katz, David L. "What if Health Were More Like Wealth?" Last modified May 9, 2012. https://www.huffpost.com/entry/health-wealth_b_1335474

Kelly, John, and Shull, Jeni. *Foundations of Lifestyle Medicine: The Lifestyle Medicine Board Review Manual, 2nd ed.* Chesterfield, MO: American College of Lifestyle Medicine, 2018.

Mayo Clinic. "Calorie Calculator." Accessed on March 5, 2022. https://www.mayoclinic.org/healthy-lifestyle/weight-loss/in-depth/calorie-calculator/itt-20402304

Laskowski, Edward R. "What Are the Risks of Sitting Too Much?" Accessed on March 5, 2022. https://www.mayoclinic.org/healthy-lifestyle/adult-health/expert-answers/sitting/faq-20058005

McGonigal, Kelly. "Here's How Exercise Reduces Anxiety and Makes You Feel More Connected." Last modified January 21, 2020. https://www.washingtonpost.com/lifestyle/2020/01/21/heres-how-exercise-reduces-anxiety-makes-you-feel-more-connected/

Miller, Rex, Williams, Phillip, and O'Neill. Michael. *The Healthy Workplace Nudge: How Healthy People, Culture, and Buildings Lead to High Performance.* Hoboken, NJ: John Wiley & Sons, 2018. Kindle.

New York Institute of Technology. "Developing Critical Thinking With Journal Writing." Accessed March 5, 2022. https://www.nyit.edu/ctl/blog/critical_thinking_journal_writing

Reeves, Mathew J., and Rafferty, Ann P. "Healthy Lifestyle Characteristics Among Adults in the United States." Arch Intern Med 165, no. 8 (2005): 854–857, https://jamanetwork.com/journals/jamainternalmedicine/fullarticle/486522

Robbins, Mel. *The 5 Second Rule: The Fastest Way to Change Your Life.* Brentwood, TN: Savio Republic, 2017. Kindle.

Sherzai, Dean, and Sherzai, Ayesha. *The 30-Day Alzheimer's Solution.* New York: HarperOne, 2021. Kindle.

Simply Psychology. "Cognitive Dissonance." Last modified February 5, 2018. https://www.simply-psychology.org/cognitive-dissonance.html

Taub-Dix, Bonnie. *Read It Before You Eat It: Taking You From Label to Table.* Self-Published, 2017. Kindle.

Terry, Bonnie. "Mind-Body Connection: Movement and Learning." Last Modified April 7, 2021. https://scholarwithin.com/mind-body-connection-movement-and-learning

Vocabulary.com. Accessed March 5, 2022. https://www.vocabulary.com/dictionary/creed

Wansink, Brian. *Slim by Design: Mindless Eating Solutions for Everyday Life.* New York: William Morrow/HarperCollins, 2014. Kindle.

www.ingramcontent.com/pod-product-compliance
Lightning Source LLC
Chambersburg PA
CBHW081325120626
46546CB00011B/3228